Starting a Healthy Lifestyle for Beginners

Nutrition & Diet Edition, Volume 1

Nancy Tran

Published by HPN, 2021.

While every precaution has been taken in the preparation of this book, the publisher assumes no responsibility for errors or omissions, or for damages resulting from the use of the information contained herein.

STARTING A HEALTHY LIFESTYLE FOR BEGINNERS

First edition. February 1, 2021.

ISBN: 979-8215624746

Written by Nancy Tran.

Table of Contents

FOREWORD 1

INTRODUCTION 2

Chapter 1: WHY HEALTHY EATING AND ITS BENEFITS 3

CHAPTER 2: WHAT DOES A HEALTHY LIFESTYLE MEAN? . 5

CHAPTER 3: DIGESTIVE HEALTH 8

Understanding Digestion: 9

Strategies for enhancing digestive health 12

Chapter 4: intermittent fasting 15

What is intermittent fasting? 16

Incorporating Intermittent Fasting into Your Life: 18

Chapter 5: detoxification 20

Understanding detoxification: 21

Improved Digestion and Gut Health: 22

Approaching Detoxification Safely: 23

Chapter 6: Superfoods: Nourishing Your Body with Nature's Powerhouse 25

Understanding Superfoods: 26

What defines a superfood? 27

Chapter 7 Berry Bonanza: Unleashing the Health Benefits of Berries 32

Berrylicious Delights: Irresistible Recipes Bursting with Berry Goodness 34

Chapter 8: Leafy Greens Powerhouse: Unveiling the Nutritional Benefits of Kale, Spinach, and Swiss Chard 38

Chapter 10: Nourishing Recipes for a Healthy Eating Journey 40

Chapter 11 Healthy Snacks for Sustained Energy and Vitality 42

Chapter 12: Nourishing Soups and Stews for Comfort and Wellness . 45

Chapter 13: Nourishing Plant-Based Meals 47

Chapter: The Power of Hydration 49

The Importance of Hydration: 50

Chapter 14: The Role of Exercise in a Healthy Lifestyle 61

Benefits of Exercise: 62

Chapter 15: The Importance of Sleep 64

Benefits of Good Sleep: 65

FINAL THOUGHTS 68

References 70

To all those who strive to live their best lives, May this book be a guiding light on your journey to health and well-being.

May it empower you with knowledge and inspire you to make positive changes. This dedication is for you as you embrace a healthy lifestyle.

May you find joy, balance, and fulfillment in nurturing your body, mind, and soul.

FOREWORD

Welcome to the first book in the "Starting a Healthy Lifestyle for Beginners" series. Here, you will discover easy, motivating, and straightforward guidelines to help you embark on a healthy eating journey.

My deep-rooted passion lies in health and wellness, and I have made these practical steps a daily ritual in my own life. This book aims to inspire and encourage people like you to embrace a healthy lifestyle.

Incorporating these simple habits into your routine will positively impact your mind, body, and soul and restore balance to your hectic daily life.

This personal journey towards healthy living has been transformative for me. It has instilled in me a profound sense of gratitude, aided in finding inner calm, and allowed me to discover true peace within myself.

I can inspire you, empowering you to live each day at your healthiest and with boundless joy.

INTRODUCTION

In our fast-paced world, convenience, fast food, and a Western diet often contain processed ingredients, chemicals, pesticides, and non-organic production methods. Unfortunately, many of us lack awareness or understanding of healthy living and struggle to find the right balance.

To address stress, anxiety, emotions, and overall well-being, I have outlined the benefits of healthy eating and created a beginner's guide to help you start your journey toward a more nutritious diet.

These guidelines will genuinely make a difference in your life. Not only will you become more conscious of what you're eating, but you will also experience deeper nourishment. Your body will efficiently digest food, leading to increased energy, enhanced cognitive function, and improved mental focus, enabling you to perform at your best.

Chapter 1: Why healthy eating and its benefits

Healthy eating brings numerous benefits, such as:

Support for local farmers: Following organic and biodynamic farming principles, farmers produce healthy, nutrient-rich food without harmful chemicals and pesticides. Organic agriculture adopts state-of-the-art farming technology to benefit the environment and grow nutritious products free from toxicity. Biodynamic farming goes further, considering all elements as interrelated living systems—animals, plants, and the planet. Biodynamic practices create healthier plants, heal the Earth by replenishing the soil, and add vitality to plants, dirt, and livestock.

Balance: Finding the right balance in all aspects of life is crucial to live well and be healthy. We must make time for work, rest, sleep, play, exercise, fresh air, family and friends, and solitude—doing everything that promotes a healthy balance. Living and eating healthily balance our mind, body, and soul.

Positive intention: The power of your mind and the impact of positive choices can significantly improve your overall health. Your mind is a powerful tool; learning to utilize it entirely is transformative. The strength of our thoughts and intentions surpasses our imagination. Increasing awareness of our food and its natural quality builds a better understanding of our bodies, eating habits, choices, and relationship with nutrition and the planet.

Well-rounded diet: Healthy eating focuses on organic and whole foods that provide all the nutrients our bodies need. It can help reduce blood pressure, which is equivalent to a decrease in stress and anxiety. The emphasis is on limiting meat, dairy products, and refined sugar, supported by ample research.

Increased energy and well-being: Consuming natural, organic, whole foods increases energy and overall well-being. Many athletes and celebrities follow a plant-based diet, which aids physical stamina, energy levels, and peak performance.

Good intestinal health: A healthy intestine forms the foundation of a healthy body, as many diseases originate in the gut. The intestinal microbiome, consisting of "good bacteria," breaks down food into readily absorbable nutrients. Imbalances in the gut have been linked to conditions such as Crohn's Disease, Ulcerative Colitis, and irritable bowel syndrome (IBS).

Environmental and animal welfare: A plant-based diet promotes health, minimizes environmental harm, and avoids animal cruelty. Plant cultivation has a lesser negative impact on the environment than animal agriculture. Organic farming, in particular, contributes to climate change mitigation by storing more carbon in the soil than non-organic methods.

By opting for organic food and being mindful of food sources, you reduce exposure to toxic chemicals and pesticides commonly used in conventional food production. Consuming meat and animal products increase your intake of dietary antibiotics, artificial hormones, industrial toxins, mercury, lead, and other heavy metals.

By making conscious choices about what you eat, you can positively impact your health, the environment, and animal.

Chapter 2: What does a healthy lifestyle mean?

A healthy lifestyle encompasses various aspects that contribute to overall well-being. It involves conscious choices regarding nutrition, sleep, physical activity, and mental health. Adopting a healthy lifestyle can maintain and improve your health while reducing the risk of numerous health conditions and promoting a sense of vitality and balance.

Nutritious Food:

One of the fundamental pillars of a healthy lifestyle is nourishing your body with nutritious food. This includes opting for organic or wholesome food whenever possible. Organic food is grown without synthetic pesticides, genetically modified organisms (GMOs), or artificial additives. Healthy food refers to unprocessed or minimally processed options that retain natural nutrients. Choosing nutrient-dense foods gives your body the essential vitamins, minerals, and antioxidants to function optimally.

Sleep:

Sufficient and restful sleep is crucial for maintaining a healthy lifestyle. Aim to get 7-8 hours of sleep each night to allow your body to rest, recover, and rejuvenate. During sleep, your body undergoes essential processes such as tissue repair, hormone regulation, and memory consolidation. Prioritizing sleep helps improve cognitive function, mood, immune function, and overall well-being.

Physical Activity:

Daily movement and exercise are integral components of a healthy lifestyle. Engaging in a combination of resistance training and cardiovascular exercises offers many benefits. Resistance training helps build and maintain muscle strength and bone density, while cardiovascular exercises improve cardiovascular health, endurance, and overall fitness. Find activities you enjoy, such as walking, jogging, swimming, dancing, or participating in sports, and strive for at least 150 minutes of moderate or 75 minutes of vigorous-intensity exercise each week.

Mental Health:

Taking care of your mental health is equally important in maintaining a healthy lifestyle. Stress management techniques, such as deep breathing exercises and meditation, can help reduce stress and anxiety and promote a sense of calm and clarity. Engaging in activities that bring you joy, such as hobbies, spending time with loved ones, practicing mindfulness, or seeking professional support, contributes to overall mental well-being.

The Benefits of a Healthy Lifestyle:

Adopting a healthy lifestyle has numerous benefits. It helps prevent overweight or obesity, tooth decay, high blood pressure, high cholesterol, heart disease, stroke, type 2 diabetes, osteoporosis, certain cancers, depression, and eating disorders. By prioritizing your health and well-being, you can improve your physical and mental resilience, enhance your immune system, increase energy levels, improve mood, and promote longevity.

Embarking on the Journey:

While committing to a healthy lifestyle may seem daunting, it is a long-term journey that becomes more comfortable with time. By building good habits gradually, one step at a time, you will find that they become second nature. Remember, taking the first step is crucial, and each subsequent step brings you closer to a healthier and more fulfilling life.

In the following chapters, we will explore practical strategies, tips, and guidelines to help you navigate the various aspects of a healthy lifestyle. From nutritious meal planning and mindful eating to effective exercise routines and stress management techniques, you will find valuable insights and actionable steps to support your journey toward a healthier and happier life.

Chapter 3: Digestive health

Understanding Digestion:

Digest begins in the mouth as food passes through the esophagus and into the stomach. It then proceeds to the small intestine, which spans approximately 20 feet long for an average person. Within the small intestine, food is broken down, and its nutrients are absorbed into the bloodstream. This breakdown allows the body to utilize the nutrients for energy, muscle building, and cell repair.

Optimizing Digestion:

It is essential to consider specific eating techniques and habits to support optimal digestion. Pairing specific foods together can enhance digestion by leveraging complementary enzymes. For example, combining proteins and carbohydrates can aid in the breakdown and assimilation of nutrients. Additionally, incorporating fresh organic vegetables (at least five servings a day) and fruit (at least two servings daily) can improve digestion due to their high water and fibre content.

The Role of Fiber:

A fibre-rich diet is vital to maintaining healthy digestion and reducing the risk of future diseases. Plant-based foods high in fibre promote healthy bowel movements and facilitate efficient transit through the intestines, minimizing fermentation and putrefaction processes.

Beneficial Probiotics:

Integrating fermented foods into your diet provides a source of beneficial probiotics. Foods such as kimchi, miso, sauerkraut, and fermented ginger contain probiotics that promote the growth of good bacteria in the intestines. Greek or coconut yogurt, kefir, and plant-based probiotics are also valuable sources of probiotics that support a healthy gut.

Negative Impact of Poor Digestion:

If your body is not digesting properly, it may indicate a diet rich in processed foods that stress the body, impede digestion, deplete nutrients, and lead to low energy levels. Processed food and red meat have been linked to digestive cancers, including liver and colon cancer. Limiting consumption of these foods or opting for healthier alternatives such as grass-fed or plant-based meats is advisable.

Enhancing Meat Digestion:

Meat can be challenging to digest due to its low fibre and water content. To aid in meat digestion, chew slowly and refrain from drinking immediately after swallowing a bite. Proper digestion prevents undigested meat from causing a toxic buildup in the intestines. Additionally, ensure that meats are adequately cooked and cleaned to minimize the risk of parasites and intestinal issues.

Making the Right Food Choices:

Being mindful of the origin of your food, particularly animal products, is crucial. Ask questions about the sources of the food you purchase and consume. Consider getting tested for food sensitivities and make dietary changes accordingly. Common allergens include gluten, dairy products, nuts, and corn. Reducing or eliminating processed foods and choosing plant-based options can significantly improve digestion. It is also advisable to reduce the consumption of caffeine, carbonated beverages, alcohol, deep-fried foods, refined sugar, non-organic soy, and meat products.

Understanding Fruit Consumption:

While fruits are rich in antioxidants, nutrients, and natural sugars (fructose), it is essential to consume them in moderation. Unripe fruits require more energy to digest. Consider the following tips when incorporating fruits into your diet:

- Consume fruits when they are ripe.

- Separate sweet and acidic fruits for better digestion.

- Include fruits as at least 15% of your daily intake.

- Due to their high sugar content, melons are best consumed separately.

- When drinking fruit juice, dilute it with 80% naturally filtered water to enhance digestibility.

- Avoid consuming fruits and vegetables together, as they require different enzymes for digestion. Simultaneous consumption may lead to bloating and gas.

By prioritizing digestive health and making mindful choices about the foods you consume, you can optimize digestion, improve nutrient absorption and support overall well-being. In the subsequent chapters, we will explore strategies and tips to enhance digestive health and incorporate these practices into daily life.

Strategies for enhancing digestive health

Taking proactive steps to enhance your digestive health can profoundly impact your well-being. In this chapter, we will explore various strategies and practical tips that you can incorporate into your daily life to optimize digestion and support a healthy gut.

Eat Mindfully:

Practicing mindful eating can significantly improve digestion. Slow down and savour each bite, thoroughly chewing your food before swallowing. Avoid rushing through meals and take the time to appreciate the flavours and textures of the food. Eating in a relaxed environment without distractions can help your body focus on digestion.

Stay Hydrated:

Adequate hydration is essential for maintaining optimal digestive function. Drink sufficient water throughout the day to support food movement through your digestive system. Aim to consume at least 8 glasses of water daily, and increase your intake during hot weather or periods of physical activity.

Increase Fiber Intake:

Fibre plays a vital role in promoting healthy digestion. Include a variety of fibre-rich foods in your diet, such as whole grains, legumes, fruits, and vegetables. These foods add bulk to your stool, facilitate regular bowel movements, and help prevent constipation. Gradually increase your fibre intake to allow your body to adjust.

Incorporate Probiotics:

Probiotics are beneficial bacteria that support a healthy gut microbiome. Consider including probiotic-rich foods, such as yogurt, kefir, sauerkraut, kimchi, and kombucha. These foods can help restore the balance of good bacteria in your digestive system and enhance nutrient absorption.

Manage Stress:

Chronic Stress can have a negative impact on digestion. Practice stress-management techniques such as deep breathing exercises, meditation, yoga, or engaging in activities that promote relaxation. Finding healthy outlets for Stress can help alleviate digestive issues such as indigestion, bloating, and discomfort.

Exercise Regularly:

Regular physical activity benefits your overall health and supports healthy digestion. Engaging in moderate exercise, such as brisk walking, swimming, or cycling, can stimulate the muscles of your digestive system, aiding in more efficient digestion and preventing constipation.

Identify Food Sensitivities:

Pay attention to how your body reacts to certain foods. Keep a food diary to track any symptoms or discomfort you experience after eating specific foods. This can help you identify food sensitivities or intolerances that may impact your digestion. Consider consulting a healthcare professional or registered dietitian/ nutritionist for further evaluation if you suspect any sensitivities.

Practice Portion Control:

Overeating can strain your digestive system and lead to discomfort—practice portion control by listening to your body's hunger and fullness cues. Eat until you are comfortably satisfied rather than overly full. Taking smaller, more frequent meals throughout the day can also aid digestion.

Avoid Trigger Foods:

Certain foods can trigger digestive issues in individuals. Pay attention to how your body reacts to common culprits such as spicy foods, fatty or greasy foods, caffeine, alcohol, and carbonated beverages. Limit or avoid these foods if they consistently cause digestive discomfort.

Seek Professional Guidance:

If you experience persistent or severe digestive issues, it is advisable to seek guidance from a healthcare professional or a registered dietitian/ nutritionist. They can provide personalized advice and recommendations based on your specific needs and help identify any underlying digestive conditions that may require further treatment.

Incorporating these strategies into your daily life can foster a healthy digestive system, improve nutrient absorption, and minimize digestive discomfort. Remember that everyone's digestion is unique, so it may take some time to identify the best approaches for you. Stay committed to your journey toward optimal digestive health, and be patient with as you make gradual adjustments to your lifestyle and dietary habits.

Chapter 4: intermittent fasting

Intermittent fasting has gained significant attention recently for its potential health benefits, including improved metabolism, enhanced focus, and overall well-being. In this chapter, we will explore the concept of intermittent fasting, its various approaches, and its potential positive effects on your body, mind, and spirit.

What is intermittent fasting?

Intermittent fasting is an eating pattern involving alternating fasting periods and eating within a specified time window. The most common approach is restricting your eating to six to eight hours, allowing your body to rest and rejuvenate during fasting. This approach can promote fat loss, improve metabolic function, and even reduce the risk of certain chronic diseases.

Types of Intermittent Fasting:

Time-Restricted Feeding:

This method restricts your daily eating to a specific time frame, typically within six to eight hours. For example, you may eat all your meals between 12 pm and 8 pm, fasting for the remaining 16 hours of the day. This approach is popular as it can be easily incorporated into daily routines.

Alternate-Day Fasting:

Alternate-Day Fasting involves alternating between fasting days and non-fasting days. On fasting days, you consume little to no calories, while on non-fasting days, you usually eat. This approach can help reduce triglyceride levels, improve LDL cholesterol, and promote overall health indicators.

Benefits of Intermittent Fasting:

Weight Loss and Metabolic Health:

Intermittent fasting can promote weight loss by reducing overall calorie intake and improving metabolic function. During fasting periods, your body relies on stored fat for energy, leading to fat loss over time. Additionally, intermittent fasting has been shown to improve insulin sensitivity and lower blood sugar levels, potentially reducing the risk of type 2 diabetes.

Increased Autophagy:

Autophagy is a cellular process that involves the recycling and renewal of damaged cells. Intermittent fasting can stimulate autophagy, which may have anti-aging and disease-fighting benefits. By promoting cellular repair and regeneration, intermittent fasting supports overall cellular health.

Cognitive Benefits:

Intermittent fasting has shown promising effects on brain health and cognitive function. It can enhance focus, concentration, and mental clarity, appealing to those seeking improved productivity and mental performance.

Reduced Inflammation and Disease Risk:

Chronic inflammation is a crucial driver of many diseases, including heart disease, cancer, and neurodegenerative conditions. Intermittent fasting has been shown to reduce inflammation markers in the body, potentially lowering the risk of developing these diseases.

Incorporating Intermittent Fasting into Your Life:

Consult a Healthcare Professional and a Nutritionist:

Before starting any fasting regimen, it's essential to consult with your healthcare professional or a nutritionist, especially if you have any underlying medical conditions or concerns. They can guide and ensure it aligns with your needs and goals.

Start Slowly:

If you're new to intermittent fasting, slowly and gradually increasing fasting periods is best. Begin with time-restricted feedings, such as an eight-hour eating window, and progressively decrease the eating window as you become accustomed to the fasting periods.

Stay Hydrated:

During fasting periods, it's crucial to stay hydrated. Drink plenty of water, herbal tea, and other non-caloric beverages to keep your body hydrated and support proper bodily functions.

Choose Nutrient-Dense Foods:

When breaking your fast, prioritize nutrient-dense foods that provide essential vitamins, minerals, and antioxidants. Focus on whole, unprocessed foods such as fruits, vegetables, lean proteins, healthy fats, and whole.

Grains nourish your body effectively.

Listen to Your Body:

Pay attention to your body's signals and adjust your fasting schedule accordingly. If you feel excessively hungry or tired, consider modifying your fasting window or seeking guidance from a healthcare professional.

Maintain a Balanced Lifestyle:

Intermittent fasting should be viewed as a tool to support a healthy lifestyle, not as a quick fix or a means to justify poor dietary choices. Combine it with regular physical activity, sufficient sleep, stress management techniques, and a well-rounded diet to optimize overall health and well-being.

Intermittent fasting offers a flexible and potentially beneficial approach to improving your health. Whether you choose time-restricted feeding or alternate-day fasting, incorporating intermittent fasting into your lifestyle requires careful consideration, gradual adjustment, and mindful eating habits. By working closely with your healthcare professional or a nutritionist and listening to your body's needs, you can harness the potential benefits of intermittent fasting and optimize your overall well-being.

Chapter 5: Detoxification

Detoxification, commonly called detox, is eliminating toxins from the body. While detoxification can encompass various aspects, including substance use detoxification, this chapter will focus on the general concept of detoxification and its potential benefits for overall health and well-being.

Understanding detoxification:

Detoxification is a natural process within our bodies to eliminate harmful substances and restore balance. Our bodies have built-in detoxification mechanisms primarily involving the liver, kidneys, lymphatic system, and skin. These systems work together to identify, neutralize, and eliminate toxins that we encounter from our environment, diet, and lifestyle choices.

The Importance of Regular Detoxification:

In today's world, where we are exposed to numerous environmental toxins and often consume processed foods, supporting our body's natural detoxification process becomes increasingly crucial. Regular detoxification can help optimize organ function, enhance immune system response, and improve overall health. While the body has its detoxification mechanisms, adopting certain practices and lifestyle changes can further support these processes and aid in eliminating toxins.

Benefits of Detoxification:

Enhanced Energy and Vitality:

Detoxification can rejuvenate the body by eliminating toxins contributing to fatigue, brain fog, and sluggishness. By reducing the toxic load, individuals often experience increased energy levels, improved mental clarity, and enhanced overall vitality.

Improved Digestion and Gut Health:

Detoxification protocols often focus on dietary modifications that support gut health. Individuals may experience improved digestion, reduced bloating, and enhanced nutrient absorption by eliminating processed foods, refined sugars, and potential food allergens.

Enhanced Immune Function:

Toxins can burden the immune system, making it less effective in fighting infections and diseases. By reducing the toxic load through detoxification, individuals can support and strengthen their immune system, leading to improved immune function and better overall health.

Clearer Skin:

Many toxins accumulate in the body and can manifest on the skin as acne, rashes, or other skin issues. Detoxification can help to improve skin health by eliminating toxins, reducing inflammation, and promoting a healthy complexion.

Weight Management:

Detoxification can assist in weight management by reducing the toxic burden on fat cells. Toxins stored in fat cells can interfere with metabolism and hinder weight loss efforts. Individuals may experience improved metabolism and better weight management outcomes by supporting the body's natural detoxification processes.

Approaching Detoxification Safely:

Consult with a Nutritionist or Healthcare Professional:

Before embarking on any detoxification program, it is essential to consult with a nutritionist or healthcare professional. They can guide you through the process, assess your specific needs, and tailor a detoxification plan that is safe and effective for you.

Choose Whole, Nutrient-Dense Foods:

During a detox, focus on consuming whole, unprocessed foods rich in nutrients. Include plenty of fruits, vegetables, lean proteins, whole grains, and healthy fats to provide your body with the essential vitamins, minerals, and antioxidants for optimal detoxification.

Stay Hydrated:

Proper hydration is vital for supporting detoxification processes. Drink adequate water throughout the day to help flush out toxins and keep your body hydrated.

Supportive Practices:

Incorporate supportive practices into your detoxification routine, such as regular exercise, stress management techniques (meditation or yoga), and sufficient sleep. These practices can further aid in the detoxification process and support overall well-being.

Gradual Transition:

Avoid sudden and drastic changes to your diet and lifestyle. Instead, ease into detoxification by gradually eliminating processed foods, refined sugars, and other potential toxins. This approach allows your body to adjust.

More comfortably and reduces the likelihood of experiencing severe detoxification symptoms.

Detoxification is a valuable practice that supports the body's natural ability to eliminate toxins and restore balance. You can safely and effectively embark on a detoxification journey by working with a nutritionist or healthcare professional, adopting a whole food-based diet, staying hydrated, and incorporating supportive practices. Regular detoxification can improve energy levels, digestion, immune function, skin health, and weight management, ultimately promoting overall health and well-being.

Chapter 6: Superfoods: Nourishing Your Body with Nature's Powerhouse

In this chapter, we will dive into the fascinating world of superfoods—nature's nutritional powerhouses offering various health benefits. These nutrient-dense foods contain vitamins, minerals, antioxidants, and other compounds that support our well-being. We will explore the unique benefits of multiple superfoods and provide creative ways to incorporate them into our daily meals, making healthy eating a delicious and enjoyable experience.

Understanding Superfoods:

What defines a superfood?

A superfood is a term used to describe foods that are exceptionally nutrient-dense and offer significant health benefits. While there is no scientific or legal definition of superfoods, they are typically packed with essential vitamins, minerals, antioxidants, and other bioactive compounds that promote optimal health and well-being. Superfoods are often rich in fibre, healthy fats, and plant-based proteins while low in calories.

What differentiates superfoods is their exceptional concentration of beneficial nutrients compared to other foods. They provide a wide range of health benefits, including boosting the immune system, supporting heart health, improving brain function, reducing inflammation, aiding in weight management, and promoting healthy aging.

Superfoods can include a variety of fruits, vegetables, whole grains, legumes, nuts, seeds, and even certain types of fish. Some commonly recognized superfoods include berries (such as blueberries and goji berries), leafy greens (like kale and spinach), fatty fish (such as salmon and sardines), nuts and seeds (like almonds and chia seeds), and whole grains (including quinoa and oats).

Incorporating superfoods into your diet can help optimize your nutritional intake and support overall well-being. However, it's important to note that superfoods offer numerous health benefits, but they should be part of a balanced and varied diet that includes a wide range of nutrient-rich foods.

The nutritional profile and health benefits of superfoods

Superfoods are known for their unique nutritional profiles and numerous health benefits. Let's explore some of the key superfoods and what makes them so beneficial:

1. Berries: Berries like blueberries, strawberries, and raspberries are rich in antioxidants, which help protect cells from damage caused by free radicals. They are also high in fibre, vitamins, and minerals, promoting heart health, supporting brain function, and boosting the immune system.

2. Leafy Greens: Vegetables like kale, spinach, and Swiss chard are nutrient powerhouses. They are packed with vitamins A, C, and K and minerals like iron and calcium. Leafy greens are known for their anti-inflammatory properties, promoting bone health, and supporting healthy digestion.

3. Fatty Fish: Fish like salmon, mackerel, and sardines are excellent sources of omega-3 fatty acids, which are beneficial for heart health and brain function. These fatty acids help reduce inflammation, lower the risk of heart disease, and support cognitive function.

4. Nuts and Seeds: Almonds, walnuts, chia seeds, and flaxseeds are rich in healthy fats, fibre, and antioxidants. They provide a good source of plant-based protein, support brain health, help lower cholesterol levels, and contribute to healthy weight management.

5. Whole Grains: Whole grains such as quinoa, oats, and brown rice are high in fibre, vitamins, and minerals. They provide sustained energy, support digestive health, and help regulate blood sugar levels. Whole grains are also linked to a reduced risk of heart disease and improved weight management.

6. Green Tea: Green tea is known for its high concentration of antioxidants, particularly catechins, associated with numerous health benefits. Green tea may improve brain function, boost metabolism, support weight loss, and reduce the risk of certain types of cancer.

Incorporating superfoods into your daily meals can help provide a wide range of nutrients, promote overall health, and reduce the risk of chronic diseases. Remember to combine superfoods with other nutritious foods and maintain a balanced diet for optimal health benefits.

Harnessing the Power of Antioxidants in Superfoods

Let's delve into the fascinating world of antioxidants and their vital role in promoting overall health and well-being. Superfoods, with their exceptional antioxidant properties, are significant in maintaining our body's equilibrium and combating oxidative stress. Let's explore how antioxidants contribute to our health and the superfoods that are particularly rich in these potent compounds.

Understanding Antioxidants:

Antioxidants help protect our cells from damage caused by harmful molecules called free radicals. Free radicals are produced naturally in the body as a by-product of various metabolic processes. Still, they can also be triggered by external factors such as pollution, smoking, and unhealthy diets. When free radicals outnumber the antioxidants in our system, they can cause oxidative stress, leading to cellular damage and an increased risk of chronic diseases.

The Benefits of Antioxidants:

Antioxidants play a crucial role in maintaining our overall health by:

Neutralizing Free Radicals: Antioxidants counteract the damaging effects of free radicals, preventing cellular damage and reducing the risk of chronic diseases like heart disease, cancer, and neurodegenerative disorders.

Anti-Inflammatory Effects: Many antioxidants exhibit anti-inflammatory properties, helping to reduce inflammation in the body. Chronic inflammation is linked to various health issues, including arthritis, obesity, and cardiovascular diseases.

Skin Health: Antioxidants can help combat the effects of aging and promote healthy skin. They protect against skin damage caused by environmental factors like UV radiation and pollution, helping to maintain a youthful and vibrant appearance.

Immune System Support: Antioxidants strengthen the immune system, promoting its ability to fight infections and diseases. They assist in reducing oxidative stress on immune cells, ensuring their optimal function.

Superfoods Rich in Antioxidants:

Several superfoods are known for their high antioxidant content, including:

- Dark Berries (blueberries, blackberries, and cherries)

- Dark Chocolate

- Green Leafy Vegetables (kale, spinach, and Swiss chard)

- Colorful Vegetables (tomatoes, bell peppers, and carrots)

- Nuts and Seeds (almonds, walnuts, and chia seeds)

- Green Tea

- Turmeric

- Citrus Fruits (oranges, lemons, and grapefruits)

- Pomegranates

Incorporating Superfoods into Your Diet:

To reap the benefits of antioxidants, it is essential to incorporate superfoods into your daily meals. This chapter will provide creative and practical ways to include these antioxidant-rich foods into your diet, ensuring you receive a diverse range of nutrients and maximize their health-promoting effects.

By harnessing the power of antioxidants in superfoods, we can protect our cells, promote overall health, and reduce the risk of chronic diseases. Incorporating antioxidant-rich foods into our daily diet is a proactive step toward achieving optimal well-being and vitality. Let's explore the various ways we can embrace these nutrient-packed superfoods and experience their positive impact on our health and longevity.

Chapter 7 Berry Bonanza: Unleashing the Health Benefits of Berries

We will dive into the world of berries and uncover the remarkable health benefits they offer. Blueberries, strawberries, raspberries, and blackberries are delicious and versatile fruits and nutritional powerhouses packed with essential vitamins, minerals, and antioxidants. Let's explore these berries' unique benefits to our health and well-being.

Nutritional Powerhouses:

Berries are low in calories and nutrients, making them an excellent addition to a balanced diet. They are rich in dietary fibre, vitamins C and K, and essential minerals such as manganese and potassium. However, the true magic lies in their unique antioxidant content, differentiating them from many other fruits.

Antioxidant Superstars:

Berries, especially blueberries, strawberries, raspberries, and blackberries, are renowned for their impressive antioxidant profiles. These antioxidants, including anthocyanins, flavonols, and resveratrol, protect our cells from oxidative stress and fight off chronic diseases. Let's explore the specific benefits of these antioxidant compounds:

1. Brain Health: The antioxidants in berries have been linked to improved brain function, memory, and cognitive abilities. They may help delay brain aging and reduce the risk of age-related conditions like Alzheimer's.

2. Heart Health: Regular consumption of berries has been associated with a reduced risk of heart disease. The antioxidants in berries help lower blood pressure, improve cholesterol levels, and promote healthy blood vessel function.

3. Cancer Prevention: The powerful antioxidants in berries have been shown to have anti-cancer properties. They help neutralize free radicals, inhibit tumour growth, and reduce inflammation, offering potential protection against various types of cancer.

4. Blood Sugar Regulation: Berries have a relatively low glycemic index, meaning they don't cause significant spikes in blood sugar levels. The fibre and antioxidants in berries can also improve insulin sensitivity, making them an excellent choice for individuals with diabetes or those aiming to manage their blood sugar levels.

5. Skin Health: The antioxidants and vitamins in berries contribute to healthy and youthful skin. They help protect against skin damage caused by UV radiation, reduce signs of aging, and promote a radiant complexion.

Incorporating Berries into Your Diet:

To enjoy the benefits of berries, including them in your daily diet is essential. Whether fresh, frozen, or dried, berries can be incorporated into various dishes and meals. From smoothies and salads to oatmeal and desserts, the possibilities are endless. This chapter will provide creative and delicious ways to incorporate berries into your meals, ensuring you savour their unique flavours and reap abundant health benefits.

Berries, including blueberries, strawberries, raspberries, and blackberries, are nature's gift to our health. Packed with antioxidants, vitamins, and minerals, these colourful fruits offer various benefits, from promoting brain and heart health to supporting cancer prevention and maintaining youthful skin. By incorporating berries into our daily diet, we can enhance our overall well-being and indulge in the sweet taste of good health. Let's unlock the potential of these little nutritional powerhouses and discover the wonders they can do for our bodies and minds.

Berrylicious Delights: Irresistible Recipes Bursting with Berry Goodness

We will explore a collection of delectable recipes that showcase berries' vibrant flavours and health benefits. From refreshing smoothies to vibrant salads and indulgent desserts, these recipes will take your culinary adventures to new heights while incorporating the nutritional powerhouse of berries. Prepare to tantalize your taste buds and nourish your body with these berrylicious delights.

Mixed Berry Smoothie Bowl:

Start your day with a burst of berry goodness with this refreshing smoothie bowl. Blend a combination of your favourite berries, such as blueberries, strawberries, and raspberries, with a splash of almond milk, a dollop of Greek yogurt, and a drizzle of honey. Top it off with a sprinkle of granola, chia seeds, and additional fresh berries for a delightful and nutritious breakfast.

Berry Spinach Salad with Goat Cheese:

Combine the sweetness of berries with the freshness of spinach in this vibrant salad. Toss together a bed of baby spinach leaves, sliced strawberries, blueberries, and raspberries. Crumble some creamy goat cheese on top for added richness. Drizzle with a light balsamic vinaigrette and garnish with toasted almonds or walnuts for a satisfying and nutrient-packed salad.

Raspberry Chia Pudding:

Indulge in a creamy and guilt-free dessert with this raspberry chia pudding. Mix chia seeds, almond milk, and a touch of maple syrup in a jar or bowl. Let it sit in the refrigerator overnight, allowing the chia seeds to absorb the liquid and create a pudding-like texture. In the morning, layer the chia pudding with fresh raspberries and top with a sprinkle of shredded coconut or crushed nuts for added crunch.

Blueberry Oatmeal Bars:

Satisfy your sweet tooth with these wholesome blueberry oatmeal bars. Combine rolled oats, almond flour, coconut oil, and a hint of honey to create a crumbly oat base. Spread a layer of blueberry compote or fresh blueberries on top and sprinkle with a streusel-like topping made from oats, almonds, and cinnamon. Bake until golden brown, and enjoy these delicious bars as a snack or dessert.

Mixed Berry Frozen Yogurt:

Cool down on a warm day with this refreshing and creamy mixed berry frozen yogurt. Blend a mix of frozen berries, such as strawberries, blackberries, and blueberries, with Greek yogurt, a squeeze of lemon juice, and a touch of honey. Pour the mixture into an ice cream maker and churn until smooth and frozen. Serve in bowls or cones and garnish with fresh mint leaves for an extra pop of freshness.

These delightful recipes featuring berries will satisfy your cravings while boosting essential nutrients and antioxidants. Whether starting your day with a vibrant smoothie bowl, enjoying a refreshing salad, indulging in a guilt-free dessert, or cooling off with homemade frozen yogurt, berries will add flavour and nutritional goodness to your meals. So, grab your apron, gather your favourite berries, and embark on a berrylicious culinary journey that will nourish your body and delight your taste buds.

Leafy Greens: Green Goodness for Vitality:

- Exploring the nutritional benefits of leafy greens like kale, spinach, and Swiss chard.

- How leafy greens contribute to detoxification, bone health, and immune function.

- Creative ways to incorporate leafy greens into everyday meals, such as green smoothies, hearty salads, and sautéed greens.

Nuts and Seeds: Tiny Packages of Nutrition:

- Unleashing the nutritional power of nuts and seeds, including almonds, walnuts, chia seeds, and flaxseeds.

- The heart-healthy fats, protein, and fibre found in nuts and seeds.

- Incorporating nuts and seeds into recipes like homemade granola bars, nut butter spreads, and nutrient-packed trail mixes.

Ancient Grains: Rediscovering Nutritional Richness:

- Exploring ancient grains like quinoa, amaranth, and millet and their unique nutritional profiles.

- The benefits of incorporating whole grains into a balanced diet include improved digestion and sustained energy levels.

- Inspiring recipes featuring ancient grains, such as quinoa salads, grain bowls, and wholesome grain-based dishes.

Plant-Based Proteins: Powering Up without Meat:

- Discovering the protein-rich options of plant-based superfoods like lentils, beans, and tofu.

- The benefits of plant-based proteins for muscle growth, weight management, and cardiovascular health.

- Delicious recipes showcasing plant-based proteins, such as lentil soups, chickpea curries, and tofu stir-fries.

Superfoods offer a treasure trove of nutritional benefits that can support our overall health and well-being. By incorporating these nutrient-dense foods into our daily meals, we can enjoy a delicious and balanced diet that nourishes our bodies from within. With the knowledge gained from this chapter, readers will be equipped to explore the world of superfoods, experiment with new recipes, and embark on a journey of vibrant health and vitality.

Chapter 8: Leafy Greens Powerhouse: Unveiling the Nutritional Benefits of Kale, Spinach, and Swiss Chard

This chapter will delve into the incredible world of leafy greens, focusing on the nutritional powerhouses: kale, spinach, and Swiss chard. These vibrant and versatile greens offer many health benefits and are a fantastic addition to any balanced diet. Get ready to discover the remarkable nutrients and unique properties that make these leafy greens exceptional for your well-being.

Kale: The Nutrient-Rich Wonder:

Learn about the abundant nutrients in kale, making it a true superfood. From its high content of vitamins, A, C, and K content to its mineral richness with calcium and iron, kale provides a nutritional boost supporting immune function, bone health, and overall vitality. Explore various cooking methods, such as sautéing, baking, or adding raw kale to salads, to enjoy its distinct flavour and reap its countless benefits.

Spinach: The Popeye's Favorite:

Uncover the remarkable health benefits of spinach, famously known as Popeye's favourite vegetable. Discover its unique iron content, which supports red blood cell production, and its abundance of folate, vitamin C, and antioxidants. Explore recipes incorporating spinach into smoothies, salads, and cooked dishes, allowing you to enjoy its mild taste while nourishing your body from the inside out.

Swiss Chard: The Colorful Delight:

Delve into the vibrant world of Swiss chard and explore its unique nutritional composition. Rich in vitamins A, K, and C, as well as magnesium and potassium, Swiss chard offers a range of health benefits, including promoting healthy digestion, supporting bone health, and aiding in blood sugar regulation. Learn creative ways to incorporate this colourful leafy green into your meals, from sautés and stir-fries to quiches and soups.

Leafy Greens Power Salad:

Indulge in a nutritious and flavorful salad featuring a kale, spinach, and Swiss chard medley. Combine these leafy greens with various colourful vegetables, such as cherry tomatoes, cucumber slices, and shredded carrots. Enhance the salad with a protein source like grilled chicken or tofu, and add a sprinkling of seeds or nuts for an extra crunch. Drizzle with a zesty lemon vinaigrette to create a satisfying and nutrient-packed meal.

Green Smoothie Boost:

Elevate your smoothie game with the rich goodness of kale, spinach, or Swiss chard. Blend a handful of leafy greens with fruits like bananas, berries, and pineapple. Add a liquid base such as almond milk or coconut water, and for an extra nutritional boost, include ingredients like chia seeds, flaxseeds, or a scoop of protein powder. Enjoy a refreshing and nutrient-dense smoothie to kickstart your day or recharge after a workout.

The leafy greens trio of kale, spinach, and Swiss chard are nutritional powerhouses offering abundant vitamins, minerals, and antioxidants. Incorporating these vibrant greens into your diet can enhance your overall well-being, from supporting immune function and bone health to promoting healthy digestion and blood sugar regulation. So, embrace the versatility of kale, spinach, and Swiss chard, and explore the numerous delicious ways to enjoy these leafy greens while reaping their remarkable health benefits.

Chapter 10: Nourishing Recipes for a Healthy Eating Journey

This chapter will explore a collection of nourishing and delicious recipes that align with your healthy eating journey. These recipes are designed to be wholesome, satisfying, and packed with nutrients to support your overall well-being. From energizing breakfast options to satisfying main dishes and guilt-free desserts, these recipes will inspire you to create nourishing and delicious meals.

1. Superfood Breakfast Bowl:

Start your day with a nutrient-packed superfood breakfast bowl. Combine a Greek or plant-based yogurt base with various toppings such as mixed berries, chia seeds, sliced almonds, and a drizzle of honey or maple syrup. Add a sprinkle of your favourite superfood powders like acai or maca to boost antioxidants and vitality.

2. Quinoa and Vegetable Stir-Fry:

Enjoy a wholesome and satisfying meal with quinoa and vegetable stir-fry. Cook quinoa according to package instructions and set aside. In a pan, sauté a colourful array of vegetables such as bell peppers, broccoli, carrots, and snow peas. Add cooked quinoa to the pan and season with soy sauce or tamari, garlic, and ginger. Toss well to combine and serve as a delicious and nutrient-rich lunch or dinner option.

3. Roasted Salmon with Lemon and Dill:

Indulge in a heart-healthy and flavorful roasted salmon dish. Preheat the oven to 375°F (190°C)—place salmon fillets on a baking sheet lined with parchment paper. Drizzle with olive oil, squeeze fresh lemon juice over the fillets, and sprinkle with chopped dill, salt, and pepper. Bake for

12-15 minutes or until the salmon is cooked through. For a complete and nourishing meal, serve with roasted vegetables or a green salad.

4. Rainbow Veggie Salad with Citrus Dressing:

Create a vibrant and nutrient-packed salad by combining a variety of colourful vegetables. Start with a bed of mixed greens or baby spinach and top with sliced cherry tomatoes, shredded carrots, cucumber slices, bell peppers, and thinly sliced red onion. Whisk together freshly squeezed citrus juice (orange or grapefruit), olive oil, a touch of honey or maple syrup, and a pinch of salt for the dressing. Drizzle the sauce over the salad for a refreshing and wholesome meal.

5. Chia Pudding Parfait:

Indulge in a guilt-free and satisfying dessert with a chia pudding parfait. In a jar or glass, layer chia pudding made with your choice of milk (almond, coconut, or dairy), chia seeds, and a touch of sweeteners such as honey or maple syrup. Top with layers of fresh berries, sliced bananas, and a sprinkle of granola or chopped nuts. Let it sit in the refrigerator for a few hours or overnight, and enjoy a creamy and nutritious treat.

These nourishing recipes showcase the diversity and deliciousness of healthy eating. From a nutrient-packed breakfast bowl to a satisfying quinoa stir-fry, a flavorful roasted salmon dish, a vibrant veggie salad, and a guilt-free chia pudding parfait, these recipes will inspire you to embrace wholesome ingredients and create meals that are both nourishing and enjoyable. Incorporating these recipes into your healthy eating journey can nourish your body and delight your taste buds, making the path to a healthier lifestyle delightful and flavorful.

Chapter 11 Healthy Snacks for Sustained Energy and Vitality

In this chapter, we will explore various healthy snack options that will keep you energized and satisfied throughout the day. These snacks are packed with nutrient-dense ingredients to boost energy while supporting overall well-being. Whether you need a mid-morning pick-me-up or an afternoon snack, these recipes keep you nourished and focused on your healthy eating journey.

1. Energy-Boosting Trail Mix:

Create your energizing trail mix by combining a blend of raw nuts and seeds such as almonds, walnuts, pumpkin seeds, and sunflower seeds. Add dried fruits like goji berries, cranberries, and apricots for a touch of natural sweetness. For an extra kick, sprinkle in dark chocolate chips or cacao nibs. Mix everything and portion it into snack-sized bags for an easy grab-and-go option.

2. Veggie Sticks with Hummus:

Slice fresh vegetables such as carrots, celery, bell peppers, and cucumber into sticks. Pair them with a homemade hummus made from chickpeas, tahini, lemon juice, garlic, and a drizzle of olive oil. The combination of crunchy veggies and creamy hummus provides a satisfying snack rich in fibre, vitamins, and minerals.

3. Greek Yogurt Parfait:

Whip up a nutritious and protein-rich Greek yogurt parfait. Layer Greek yogurt with various toppings such as fresh berries, sliced banana, granola, and a drizzle of honey or maple syrup. For added texture and flavour, sprinkle in some crushed nuts or seeds. This snack is delicious and provides a good balance of macronutrients to keep you satiated.

4. Baked Sweet Potato Chips:

Satisfy your craving for something crispy with homemade baked sweet potato chips. Slice sweet potatoes into thin rounds, toss them in olive oil, sprinkle with sea salt and your favourite spices (such as paprika or cinnamon), and bake in the oven until crispy. Enjoy these guilt-free chips as a healthier alternative to traditional potato chips.

5. Green Smoothie:

Revitalize your body with a refreshing and nutrient-packed green smoothie. Blend a handful of leafy greens (such as spinach or kale), a ripe banana, a cup of your favourite frozen fruits (such as mango or pineapple), a scoop of plant-based protein powder, and a liquid of your choice (such as almond milk or coconut water). Blend until smooth, and enjoy this green goodness packed with vitamins, minerals, and antioxidants.

6. Homemade Energy Bars: Make your energy bars using a combination of oats, nuts, seeds, and dried fruits. Mix these ingredients with nut butter, honey, and a pinch of salt. Press the mixture into a baking dish and refrigerate until firm. Cut into bars and store them for quick and convenient snacks. These homemade energy bars contain nutrients, fibre, and natural sweetness without added preservatives or artificial ingredients.

7. Avocado Toast: Toast a slice of whole-grain bread with mashed avocado. Sprinkle with a pinch of sea salt and black pepper. Add toppings like sliced tomatoes, a squeeze of lemon juice, or a sprinkle of chia seeds for extra flavour. Avocado toast is a satisfying snack that provides healthy fats, fibre, and a range of essential vitamins and minerals.

8. Roasted Chickpeas: Roast canned or cooked chickpeas with olive oil and your choice of spices like paprika, cumin, or chilli powder. Bake

them in the oven until crispy and golden. Roasted chickpeas are a crunchy and high-fibre snack that offers a satisfying combination of protein and carbohydrates.

9. Rice Cake with Nut Butter and Berries: Spread your favourite nut butter (almond or cashew butter) onto a rice cake and top it with fresh berries like strawberries, blueberries, or raspberries. This snack is a delightful combination of textures and flavours, balancing carbohydrates, healthy fats, and antioxidants.

These healthy snack recipes offer a range of options to keep you fueled and nourished throughout the day. From an energy-boosting trail mix to veggie sticks with hummus, a Greek yogurt parfait, baked sweet potato chips, and a refreshing green smoothie, these snacks are delicious and packed with nutrients. By incorporating these recipes into your daily routine, you can maintain sustained energy levels, support your overall well-being, and stay on track with your healthy eating goals. Enjoy these snacks as a tasty and nutritious addition to your healthy lifestyle.

Chapter 12: Nourishing Soups and Stews for Comfort and Wellness

In this chapter, we will explore a variety of nourishing soup and stew recipes that provide comfort and support your overall well-being. These recipes are filled with wholesome ingredients, rich flavours, and ample nutrients to satisfy and nourish you. From hearty vegetable soups to protein-packed stews, these recipes will warm your body and nourish your soul.

1. Hearty Lentil Soup:

Start with a base of sautéed onions, garlic, and carrots. Add red lentils, vegetable broth, diced tomatoes, and a medley of cumin, turmeric, and paprika. Let the soup simmer until the tender lentils and the flavours meld together. Serve with a squeeze of lemon juice and fresh cilantro for freshness. This protein and fibre-rich soup will keep you satisfied and nourished.

2. Creamy Roasted Butternut Squash Soup:

Roast butternut squash until tender and blend it with vegetable broth, onions, garlic, and a hint of nutmeg. For added creaminess, stir in some coconut milk or cashew cream. Season with salt and pepper to taste. This velvety soup is packed with vitamins, minerals, and antioxidants, and its rich flavour is perfect for cozy evenings.

3. Chicken and Vegetable Stew:

Combine diced chicken breast, chopped onions, carrots, celery, and potatoes in a large pot. Add in low-sodium chicken broth, thyme, rosemary, and bay leaves. Let the stew simmer until the chicken is cooked and the vegetables tender. The result is a comforting and protein-packed stew that will warm you up from the inside out.

4. Quinoa and Vegetable Chili:

In a large pot, sauté onions, bell peppers, and garlic until softened. Add in diced tomatoes, black beans, kidney beans, cooked quinoa, and a blend of chilli powder, cumin, and smoked paprika. Let the chilli simmer for about 30 minutes to allow the flavours to meld together. This hearty and fibre-rich chilli is delicious and packed with plant-based protein.

5. Mushroom Barley Soup:

Sauté a mix of mushrooms, onions, and garlic until the mushrooms release their juices. Add vegetable broth, pearl barley, carrots, celery, and thyme. Simmer until the barley is tender, and the flavours have infused into the soup. This hearty and earthy soup is an excellent source of fibre, vitamins, and minerals.

These nourishing soup and stew recipes provide comfort, flavour, and a wealth of nutrients. From the hearty lentil soup to the creamy roasted butternut squash soup, chicken and vegetable stew, quinoa and vegetable chilli, and mushroom barley soup, these recipes offer various options to suit different preferences. By incorporating these recipes into your meal rotation, you can enjoy delicious and nourishing meals that support your overall wellness. Embrace the warmth and comfort of these soups and stews, and savour the goodness they bring to your table.

Chapter 13: Nourishing Plant-Based Meals

Plant-based meals are not only nutritious but also have a positive impact on your health and the environment. This chapter will explore a range of nourishing plant-based meal ideas packed with vegetables, whole grains, legumes, and plant-based proteins. These meals are delicious, promote overall well-being, and support a sustainable lifestyle.

1. Rainbow Buddha Bowl:

Create a vibrant and nourishing Buddha bowl by combining a variety of colourful vegetables such as roasted sweet potatoes, sautéed kale, shredded purple cabbage, sliced avocado, and cherry tomatoes. Add a scoop of cooked quinoa or brown rice for a satisfying grain base. Drizzle with a flavorful dressing like tahini or lemon vinaigrette for added taste. This bowl provides a wide range of nutrients, including fibre, vitamins, minerals, and antioxidants.

2. Lentil Curry:

Prepare a hearty and flavorful lentil curry by simmering lentils with aromatic spices like cumin, turmeric, and garam masala. Add diced tomatoes, onion, garlic, and ginger for a rich base. Serve the curry over a bed of fluffy basmati rice or with whole-grain naan bread. Lentils are a great source of plant-based protein, fibre, and essential minerals, making this curry nutritious and satisfying.

3. Veggie Stir-Fry:

Stir-fries are quick, versatile, and perfect for incorporating a variety of vegetables. Sauté a mix of colourful vegetables such as bell peppers, broccoli, carrots, snap peas, and mushrooms in a hot wok or skillet. Add a flavorful sauce made with soy sauce, ginger, garlic, and a touch of honey or maple syrup. Serve the stir-fry over a bed of brown rice or noodles for a complete and nourishing meal.

4. Chickpea Salad Wraps:

Make a refreshing and protein-packed chickpea salad by mashing chickpeas with diced cucumber, cherry tomatoes, red onion, and fresh herbs like parsley and cilantro. Add a squeeze of lemon juice and olive oil, drizzle, and season with salt and pepper. Spoon the chickpea salad into whole-grain wraps and garnish with avocado slices or sprouts. These wraps are a delicious and filling option for a quick and satisfying lunch or dinner.

5. Roasted Vegetable Quinoa Bowl:

Roast a medley of seasonal vegetables like Brussels sprouts, butternut squash, and cauliflower with olive oil, salt, and pepper until golden and tender. Serve the roasted vegetables over a bed of fluffy quinoa and top with toasted nuts or seeds for added crunch. Drizzle with a tangy balsamic glaze or tahini dressing for extra flavour. This wholesome bowl provides a good balance of carbohydrates, fibre, and vitamins from vegetables and quinoa.

Nourishing plant-based meals offer various flavours, textures, and nutrients, contributing to overall health and well-being. By incorporating colourful and nutrient-rich options like rainbow Buddha bowls, lentil curry, veggie stir-fries, chickpea salad wraps, and roasted vegetable quinoa bowls into your meal rotation, you can enjoy the benefits of plant-based eating while savouring delicious and satisfying meals. Whether you embrace an entirely plant-based lifestyle or incorporate more plant-based meals into your diet, these recipes nourish your body and support your health goals.

Chapter: The Power of Hydration

Water is essential for life and crucial in maintaining optimal health. In this chapter, we will delve into the importance of hydration and its impact on various aspects of well-being. From understanding the benefits of staying hydrated to exploring creative ways to enhance water intake, you will discover the power of hydration and its transformative effects on your body and mind.

The Importance of Hydration:

Water is an essential component of the human body, and its role goes far beyond simply quenching thirst. Understanding the vital functions of water in the body can help you appreciate its importance and prioritize proper hydration for overall well-being. Here are some key roles that water plays in maintaining optimal bodily functions:

1. Regulating Body Temperature:

Water is crucial for regulating body temperature, primarily through sweating and evaporation. When the body gets too hot, sweat evaporates from the skin's surface, cooling the body down. This thermoregulation mechanism helps prevent overheating and ensures the body maintains a stable internal temperature.

2. Aiding Digestion:

Water plays a vital role in Digestion and the absorption of nutrients. It helps dissolve and transport nutrients, allowing them to be absorbed by the cells in the digestive system. Water also softens stools, promoting regular bowel movements and preventing constipation.

3. Promoting Nutrient Absorption:

Water facilitates the absorption of essential nutrients, such as vitamins, minerals, and electrolytes, in the digestive tract. These nutrients are necessary for various bodily functions, including energy production, immune system support, and cellular repair.

4. Lubricating Joints:

Water helps lubricate joints, providing cushioning and reducing friction between bones. Proper hydration ensures the joints remain well-lubricated, promoting smooth and pain-free movement.

5. Supporting Overall Cellular Function:

Water is a fundamental component of all cells in the body. It helps create an optimal environment for cellular processes, including metabolism, nutrient transport, and waste removal. Water also aids in the proper functioning of the body's organs, tissues, and systems.

It's important to note that individual water needs can vary based on age, sex, activity level, and environmental conditions. Staying adequately hydrated by drinking water and consuming hydrating foods is essential for supporting these vital functions and maintaining overall health and well-being. Remember to listen to your body's thirst cues and drink water throughout the day to ensure proper hydration.

Understand the signs and symptoms of dehydration and the potential health risks associated with chronic dehydration.

Dehydration occurs when the body loses more fluid than it takes in, leading to an imbalance in the body's water levels. It's crucial to be aware of the signs and symptoms of dehydration to recognize and address it promptly. Additionally, chronic dehydration, which is a long-term condition of inadequate fluid intake, can have detrimental effects on health. Here's an overview of the signs, symptoms, and risks associated with dehydration:

Signs and Symptoms of Dehydration:

1. Increased Thirst: Feeling excessively thirsty is often the first indication of dehydration. It's your body's way of signalling that it needs more fluids.

2. Dry Mouth and Lips: Inadequate fluid intake can result in a dry mouth and parched lips. Saliva production decreases when the body is dehydrated.

3. Dark-Colored Urine: When dehydrated, your urine becomes more concentrated and darker. Ideally, urine should be a pale yellow or clear.

4. Fatigue and Weakness: Dehydration can lead to feelings of fatigue, weakness, and a lack of energy. Your body's cells require proper hydration to function optimally.

5. Dizziness and Light-headedness: Insufficient fluid levels can cause dizziness and light-headedness, as reduced blood volume affects circulation and blood flow to the brain.

6. Headaches: Dehydration can trigger headaches or migraines in some individuals. It's essential to stay hydrated to help prevent or alleviate these symptoms.

Health Risks of Chronic Dehydration:

Impaired Physical Performance: Dehydration can negatively impact physical performance, reducing endurance, muscle cramps, and decreased strength.

Kidney Problems: Chronic dehydration can contribute to the formation of kidney stones and increase the risk of urinary tract infections.

Digestive Issues: Inadequate hydration can result in constipation, as water is essential for softening stools and maintaining regular bowel movements.

Heat-Related Illnesses: Dehydration increases the risk of heat exhaustion and heat stroke, particularly in hot and humid conditions.

Impaired Cognitive Function: Studies have shown that even mild dehydration can impair cognitive function, including memory, attention, and overall mental performance.

To prevent dehydration, it's essential to drink adequate fluids throughout the day, especially during periods of physical activity, hot weather, or illness. Aim to consume water regularly and include hydrating foods, such as fruits and vegetables, in your diet. Being mindful of the signs of dehydration and prioritizing hydration can help maintain optimal health and well-being.

Optimal Water Intake:

Discover how much water you should drink each day and the factors that can influence your hydration needs, such as climate, physical activity, and overall health.

Determining how much water you should drink daily is influenced by various factors, including climate, physical activity levels, and overall health. While there is no one-size-fits-all answer, here's a general guideline to help you understand your hydration needs:

1. The 8x8 Rule suggests drinking eight 8-ounce glasses of water per day, totalling about 2 litres or half a gallon. It's a simple guideline that is easy to remember but may only be suitable for some.

2. Body Weight: Another approach is to consider your body weight. Generally, you should consume about 0.5 to 1 ounce (15 to 30 millilitres) of water per pound (0.5 to 1 millilitre per gram) of body weight. For example, if you weigh 150 pounds (68 kilograms), you would aim for 75 to 150 ounces (2.2 to 4.4 litres) of water daily.

3. Climate and Environment: Hot and humid climates can increase water loss through sweating, making it necessary to drink more fluids to maintain proper hydration. Similarly, high-altitude environments can contribute to increased water loss through respiration and may require higher fluid intake.

4. Physical Activity: Exercise or strenuous physical activity increases water loss through sweating. It's crucial to replenish fluids before, during, and after exercise. Aim to drink additional water based on the intensity and duration of your workouts.

5. Overall Health and Medical Conditions: Certain medical conditions, such as kidney stones or urinary tract infections, may require higher fluid intake to promote proper kidney function and urinary flow. Pregnant or breastfeeding women also have increased hydration needs.

Remember that these are general guidelines, and individual hydration needs can vary. Age, metabolism, and medications can influence your water requirements. Listening to your body and paying attention to thirst cues is essential. Additionally, consuming hydrating foods and beverages, such as fruits, vegetables, and herbal teas, can improve your overall hydration.

Suppose you need more clarity about your specific hydration needs or have any underlying health conditions. In that case, it's advisable to consult with a healthcare professional or registered dietitian/nutritionist who can provide personalized guidance tailored to your circumstances.

Explore different hydration guidelines and recommendations from reputable sources and health professionals/nutritionists.

Hydration guidelines and recommendations can vary based on different sources and health professionals. It's always a good idea to consult reputable sources and seek advice from qualified healthcare professionals or registered dietitians/ nutritionists for personalized recommendations. Here are some commonly referenced hydration guidelines:

1. The National Academies of Sciences, Engineering, and Medicine: The general recommendation from this organization suggests a daily water intake of about 3.7 litres (125 ounces) for men and 2.7 litres (91 ounces) for women, including fluids from all sources (beverages and foods).

2. European Food Safety Authority (EFSA): The EFSA recommends a total water intake of 2.5 litres (84 ounces) for men and 2.0 litres (68 ounces) for women, which includes fluid from beverages and food. They suggest that about 70-80% of the total water intake should come from drinks, while the remaining 20-30% can come from food.

3. Institute of Medicine (IOM): The IOM suggests a general guideline of 3.7 litres (125 ounces) for men and 2.7 litres (91 ounces) for women, including fluids from all sources.

4. American College of Sports Medicine (ACSM): The ACSM provides specific guidelines for hydration during exercise. They recommend consuming 16-20 ounces (500-600 millilitres) of fluid 4 hours before exercise, 8-12 ounces (240-360 millilitres) of juice 10-15 minutes before training, and 7-10 ounces (200-300 millilitres) of fluid every 10-20 minutes during exercise.

Remember, these guidelines are general recommendations that may only suit some. Age, body size, activity level, climate, and health conditions can influence individual hydration needs. It's essential to listen to your body's thirst cues, monitor urine colour (pale yellow generally indicates adequate hydration), and adjust your fluid intake accordingly.

Suppose you have specific concerns or medical conditions that affect your hydration needs. In that case, it's recommended to consult with a healthcare professional or registered dietitian/ nutritionist who can provide personalized advice based on your circumstances.

Hydrating Foods:

Explore a variety of hydrating foods that can contribute to your overall fluid intakes, such as fruits like watermelon and oranges, vegetables like cucumbers and celery, and soups or broths. Learn about their high-water content and additional nutritional benefits that support hydration.

Hydrating foods can play a significant role in meeting your daily fluid intake goals. Here are some examples of hydrating foods and their additional nutritional benefits:

1. Watermelon: Watermelon is composed of about 92% water, making it a fantastic choice for hydration. It's also rich in vitamins A and C and lycopene, an antioxidant that may promote heart health.

2. Oranges: Oranges are hydrating and packed with vitamin C, fibre, and antioxidants. They provide a refreshing burst of citrus flavour and can be enjoyed as a snack or squeezed into fresh juice.

3. Cucumbers: Cucumbers are incredibly hydrating, consisting of approximately 95% water. They also contain electrolytes like potassium and magnesium and vitamins K and C. Adding cucumber slices to salads or infusing water with cucumber can enhance both flavour and hydration.

4. Celery: With a high-water content of about 95%, celery is a hydrating vegetable with dietary fibre, vitamins A, K, and C, and antioxidants. It's a crunchy and refreshing addition to salads, soups, or as a snack with a healthy dip.

5. Soups and broths: Soups and broths can provide hydration and nourishment. Whether it's a vegetable-based soup or a warm bone broth, these liquids contribute to your overall fluid intake while providing additional nutrients like vitamins, minerals, and amino acids.

6. Strawberries: Strawberries have a water content of around 91% and are loaded with vitamins C and A, dietary fibre, and antioxidants. They make a delicious addition to smoothies and salads or are enjoyed as a sweet and hydrating snack.

7. Pineapple: Pineapple is hydrating and offers bromelain, an enzyme that aids digestion. It's a tropical fruit rich in vitamin C, manganese, and

antioxidants. Enjoy pineapple chunks as a refreshing snack, or add them to fruit salads and smoothies.

Incorporating these hydrating foods into your diet can provide a flavorful way to increase your fluid intake while benefiting from their additional nutritional value. Remember that hydration depends not solely on water intake but can also be obtained through beverages and hydrating foods.

Infused Water:

Discover the refreshing and flavorful world of infused water. Explore various combinations of fruits, herbs, and vegetables that can be added to water to enhance its taste and provide additional health benefits. From citrus-infused water to cucumber-mint or strawberry-basil concoctions, infused water can make hydration more enjoyable and enticing.

Infused water is a delightful way to stay hydrated while enjoying the natural flavours and benefits of fruits, herbs, and vegetables. Here are some refreshing combinations to try:

1. Citrus Burst: Add lemon, lime, and orange slices to a water pitcher. This citrus infusion provides a burst of vitamin C and adds a tangy flavour to your water.

2. Berry Bliss: Combine fresh strawberries, blueberries, and raspberries in water. Berries are rich in antioxidants and add a subtle sweetness to your infused water.

3. Cucumber Mint Cooler: Slice cucumbers and add a few sprigs of fresh mint to the water. This combination is incredibly refreshing, aids digestion, and gives a cooling effect.

4. Tropical Paradise: Create a tropical vibe by adding pineapple chunks and a squeeze of lime to your water. Pineapple is known for its digestive enzymes, while lime adds a zesty twist.

5. Watermelon Basil Splash: Blend fresh watermelon chunks with a handful of basil leaves, and mix it with water. Watermelon hydrates and replenishes electrolytes, while basil adds a hint of herbaceousness.

6. Cinnamon Apple Infusion: Slice apples and add a cinnamon stick to water. Cinnamon has potential health benefits, such as supporting blood sugar control, while apples add natural sweetness.

7. Refreshing Herb Medley: Combine rosemary, thyme, and sage sprigs in water. These herbs infuse the water with a subtle earthy aroma and provide potential antioxidant properties.

Add your chosen combination of fruits, herbs, or vegetables to a pitcher or bottle of water to prepare infused water. Allow it to sit for a few hours or overnight in the refrigerator to allow the flavours to infuse. Feel free to experiment with different combinations and adjust the intensity of flavours to suit your taste preferences.

Infused water is a tasty alternative to plain water and encourages increased water intake by making hydration more enjoyable. It's a perfect way to stay refreshed and reap the benefits of natural ingredients.

Hydration Tips and Tricks:

Get practical tips and tricks for staying hydrated throughout the day, such as carrying a reusable water bottle, setting reminders to drink water, incorporating hydrating beverages like herbal teas or coconut water, and tracking your water intake. These strategies will help you establish healthy hydration habits and make drinking enough water a seamless part of your routine.

Staying hydrated throughout the day is essential for maintaining optimal health and well-being. Here are some practical tips and tricks to help you stay hydrated:

1. Carry a reusable water bottle: Invest in a reusable water bottle you can take wherever you go. Having easy access to water will be a constant reminder to stay hydrated.

2. Set reminders: Use your phone or other devices to set reminders at regular intervals throughout the day to drink water. This will help you establish a routine and prevent dehydration.

3. Infuse your water: As mentioned earlier, infusing water with fruits, herbs, or vegetables can make it more appealing and flavorful. Experiment with different combinations to keep your taste buds engaged.

4. Drink herbal teas: Herbal teas are hydrating and offer various health benefits. Add herbal teas like chamomile, peppermint, or hibiscus to your routine to increase fluid intake.

5. Include hydrating foods: Consume high water content, such as watermelon, cucumbers, tomatoes, and leafy greens. These foods can contribute to your overall hydration while providing essential nutrients.

6. Monitor your water intake: Use a water tracking app or keep a journal to track your daily water intake. This will help you stay accountable and meet your hydration goals.

7. Sip on coconut water: Coconut water is a natural hydrator packed with electrolytes. It can be a refreshing alternative to plain water and help replenish your body's electrolyte balance.

8. Make water more appealing: If you struggle with drinking plain water, add a splash of lemon or lime juice for flavour. You can also drink water at different temperatures, such as warm or cold, to make it more enjoyable.

Everyone's hydration needs may vary depending on activity level, climate, and health conditions. Listen to your body and drink water whenever you feel thirsty. By incorporating these tips into your daily routine, you'll develop healthier hydration habits and ensure your body receives the hydration it needs to function optimally.

Hydration is a cornerstone of well-being and should be prioritized daily. By understanding the importance of hydration, optimizing your water intake, incorporating hydrating foods, experimenting with infused water, and implementing hydration tips and tricks, you can experience the transformative effects of staying adequately hydrated. Embrace the power of hydration and unlock its potential to enhance your overall health, energy levels, and vitality. Stay refreshed, rejuvenated, and hydrated for a vibrant and thriving life.

Chapter 14: The Role of Exercise in a Healthy Lifestyle

In this chapter, we will explore the significant role of exercise in maintaining a healthy lifestyle. Regular physical activity has numerous benefits for both our physical and mental well-being. We will delve into the positive effects of exercise on cardiovascular health, weight management, energy levels, and mood. Additionally, we will provide practical tips and strategies to help you incorporate exercise into your daily life.

Benefits of Exercise:

Improved Cardiovascular Health: Regular physical activity strengthens the heart and improves blood circulation, reducing the risk of cardiovascular diseases such as heart disease, stroke, and high blood pressure.

Weight Management: Exercise plays a crucial role in weight management by increasing calorie expenditure and promoting the development of lean muscle mass. Combined with a healthy diet, exercise can help maintain a healthy weight or support weight loss efforts.

Increased Energy Levels: Regular physical activity boosts energy levels by enhancing blood flow and oxygen delivery to muscles, improving endurance, and promoting better sleep quality.

Enhanced Mood and Mental Well-being: Exercise has powerful effects on mental health, stimulating the release of endorphins, often called "feel-good" hormones. It can reduce symptoms of stress, anxiety, and depression while promoting overall mental well-being.

Incorporating Exercise into Daily Life:

Find Activities You Enjoy: Choose physical activities like walking, dancing, cycling, swimming, or playing a sport. This will increase your motivation to exercise regularly.

Set Realistic Goals: Start with small, achievable goals and gradually increase the intensity and duration of your workouts. This approach will help you stay motivated and prevent injury.

Schedule Exercise: Treat exercise as an essential appointment in your daily routine. Block out specific times for physical activity and make it a priority.

Make it Social: Exercise with friends, family or join group classes. Exercising with others can make the experience more enjoyable and help you stay accountable.

Stay Active Throughout the Day: Look for opportunities to be active throughout the day, such as taking the stairs instead of the elevator, going for short walks during breaks, or incorporating physical activity into household chores.

Mix Up Your Routine: Avoid boredom by varying your exercise routine. Try different activities and alternate between cardiovascular exercises, strength training, and flexibility exercises to work for other muscle groups and keep your workouts interesting.

Regular exercise is a cornerstone of a healthy lifestyle, offering numerous physical and mental health benefits. By incorporating physical activity into your daily routine and adopting a mindset of consistency and enjoyment, you can experience the transformative power of exercise and improve your overall well-being. Start small, stay committed, and embrace the positive changes that exercise brings.

Chapter 15: The Importance of Sleep

This chapter will delve into the crucial role of quality sleep in maintaining overall health and well-being. Sleep is a fundamental physiological need in various aspects of our lives. We will explore the benefits of good sleep, the potential consequences of sleep deprivation, and provide practical strategies for improving sleep hygiene.

Benefits of Good Sleep:

Physical Health: Quality sleep is essential for optimal physical health. It supports the immune system, promotes proper hormone regulation, and aids in the repair and restoration of tissues and cells. Adequate sleep has been linked to a lower risk of chronic conditions such as obesity, diabetes, cardiovascular disease, and immune disorders.

Mental Well-being: Sleep profoundly impacts mental health and cognitive function. It enhances memory consolidation, promotes learning, and improves problem-solving abilities. Sufficient sleep also contributes to emotional regulation, reducing the risk of mood disorders such as depression and anxiety.

Energy and Productivity: Quality sleep is directly linked to increased energy levels, alertness, and productivity. When well-rested, we experience improved focus, concentration, and mental clarity, allowing us to perform at our best in daily tasks and responsibilities.

Consequences of Sleep Deprivation:

Impaired Cognitive Function: Lack of sleep can lead to difficulties in concentration, memory problems, reduced attention span, and impaired decision-making abilities. It can also hinder creativity and problem-solving skills.

Emotional Disturbances: Sleep deprivation can increase irritability, mood swings, and emotional instability. It may contribute to heightened stress levels, anxiety, and an increased risk of developing mental health disorders.

Weakened Immune System: Inadequate sleep weakens the immune system, making us more susceptible to infections, viruses, and chronic illnesses. It also reduces the body's ability to recover from illness or injury.

Improving Sleep Hygiene:

Establish a Consistent Sleep Schedule: Aim to go to bed and wake up simultaneously every day, even on weekends. This helps regulate your body's internal clock and promotes better sleep quality.

Create a Relaxing Bedtime Routine: Engage in calming activities before bed, such as reading, taking a warm bath, practicing relaxation techniques, or listening to soothing music. Avoid stimulating activities or bright screens close to bedtime.

Create a Sleep-Friendly Environment: Make sure your sleep environment is comfortable, quiet, dark, and relaxed. Use comfortable bedding and invest in a supportive mattress and pillow. Consider using white noise machines or earplugs if noise is an issue.

Limit Stimulants and Electronic Devices: Avoid consuming caffeine, nicotine, and alcohol close to bedtime, as they can disrupt sleep patterns. Additionally, minimize screen time before bed, as the blue light emitted by electronic devices can interfere with melatonin production.

Engage in Regular Physical Activity: Regular exercise during the day can promote better sleep quality. However, avoid intense exercise close to bedtime, as it can be stimulating.

Quality sleep is a vital component of overall health and well-being. You can prioritize and improve your sleep hygiene by understanding the benefits of good sleep and the potential consequences of sleep deprivation. Incorporating practical strategies such as maintaining a consistent sleep schedule, creating a relaxing bedtime routine, and optimizing your sleep environment can help you achieve restful and rejuvenating sleep. Make sleep a priority and experience its positive impact on your physical health, mental well-being, and daily productivity.

FINAL THOUGHTS

Congratulations on reaching the end of this book! I express my sincere gratitude for taking the time to read and explore the world of healthy eating. Investing in your well-being is a significant step towards a healthier and happier life.

Remember, healthy eating is not a daunting task. It is an attainable goal that begins with prioritizing your health. As you embark on this journey, I encourage you to approach it with determination and a positive mindset. Taking care of yourself is a worthwhile investment that will benefit your body, mind, and soul in the long run.

Cooking can be more than just a necessary task; it can also be a therapeutic and enjoyable experience. Whether preparing meals for yourself or sharing them with loved ones, cooking and sharing nourishing food creates a sense of joy and connection.

If you require personalized guidance on your health journey, I offer 1-on-1 consultations to develop customized health plans. These consultations will help you create a roadmap toward your specific health goals, addressing your unique needs and preferences.

Please share your experience with this book by leaving a review on Google or Facebook or providing a testimonial on my website at www.holisticpharmacyandnutrition.com. Your feedback and thoughts will help others discover the benefits of healthy eating and make informed decisions about their well-being.

If you have any further questions or require additional assistance, please don't hesitate to contact me via email at hpnnutrition@gmail.com. I am here to support you on your journey toward a healthier lifestyle.

Thank you once again for your time and commitment to your health. I wish you abundant health, happiness, and fulfillment.

With warm regards,

Nancy Tran

Registered Holistic Nutritionist & Certified Strength and Conditioning Specialist

References

New Year, New Wellness - Country Roads Magazine. https://countryroadsmagazine.com/art-and-culture/people-places/new-year-new-wellness-pennington/

55 Hobbies for Men of All Ages. https://www.developgoodhabits.com/hobbies-men/

About - Yogananda Association. https://yogananda-association.org/ya-about/

Meditation for Beginners – Bonafide. https://hellobonafide.com/blogs/news/meditation-for-beginners

Journal – Byome. https://thebyome.com/blogs/journal

Best Way to Lose Weight | Find It And Share It. http://finditandshareit.com/best-way-to-lose-weight/

Our organic and sustainable farm • Somnatur. https://www.somnatur.com/nosotros

7 Natural Ways to Boost Your Immune System and Stay Healthy – Upper Valley Artist & Farmers Market. https://uppervalleymarket.com/blogs/upper-valley-market-blogs/7-natural-ways-to-boost-your-immune-system-and-stay-healthy

How can I remove pimples to my face? – drpopr. https://drpopr.com/index.php/2023/01/15/how-can-i-remove-pimples-to-my-face/

4 Essential Exercises to Keep You Feeling Young as You Age – The Abundance Pub. https://theabundancepub.com/4-essential-exercises-to-keep-you-feeling-young-as-you-age/

These 5 Things Will Help You Live Longer - YoTrending. https://yotrending.com/these-5-things-will-help-you-live-longer/

Scottsdale Public Library - Young Adult Books. https://www.scottsdalelibrary.org/teen/books

8 Simple Ways to Boost Testosterone Levels – Agent Steel Online. https://www.agentsteelonline.com/8-simple-ways-to-boost-testosterone-levels/

The benefits of incorporating mindfulness and meditation into your fitness routine - The Channel 46: Uncomplicating Health and Beauty For Indian Women. https://www.thechannel46.com/web-stories/the-benefits-of-incorporating-mindfulness-and-meditation-into-your-fitness-routine/

Emerald City | Lo Bou. https://www.shoplobou.com/product-page/emerald-city

Building resilience in your recovery | EPIC Restart Foundation. https://www.epicrestartfoundation.org/articles/building-resiliance-in-your-recovery

Advanced Nutritional Test - SYNLAB Nigeria. https://www.synlab.com.ng/info-page/nutrihealth/

The 10 ideal healthy lifestyle for adults (What you need to maximize your health). https://lodpost.com/the-10-ideal-healthy-lifestyle-for-adults-what-you-need-to-maximize-your-health-9485

Get in shape | EUTF | Kaiser Permanente. https://mybenefits.kaiserpermanente.org/eutf/get-in-shape

From diverticulosis to diverticulitis: Prof. Danese on TV2000 - Humanitas.net. https://www.humanitas.net/news/diverticulosis-diverticulitis-prof-danese-tv2000/

5 Simple Ways To Lower Your Electricity Bill - Practical Smart. https://practicalsmart.com/5-simple-ways-to-lower-your-electricity-bill/

5 ways to incorporate mindfulness into your everyday life – Improving Slowly. https://improvingslowly.com/2019/10/12/5-ways-to-incorporate-mindfulness-into-your-everyday-life/

Water – Drink Up! – Shape180. https://shape180fitness.com/2013/10/16/water-drink-up/

Weight Loss Tips - Glow Bar London. https://glowbarldn.com/blogs/cbd-guides/weight-loss-tips

Probiotics for Dogs: Uses, Benefits, and Precautions | Daily Paws. https://www.dailypaws.com/dogs-puppies/health-care/dog-medications/probiotics-for-dogs

Tips For Staying Healthy And Active As You Age - Ageful. https://www.ageful.com/tips-for-staying-healthy-and-active-as-you-age/

.   https://www.seniorhelpers.com/fl/pasco-west/resources/blogs/8-new-years-resolutions-for-caregivers-of-senior-parents/

Irish do less exercise than Americans · TheJournal.ie. https://www.thejournal.ie/irish-do-less-exercise-than-americans-524821-Jul2012/

Lets talk about Caffine in your Fyngan cup of coffee. https://fyngan.com/blogs/speciality-coffee/lets-talk-about-caffine-in-your-coffee

Certified Health Coach Analee Joseph helps people embark on their journey toward body transformation with Optavia-powered diet plans – Rainbownewsline. http://news.rainbownewsline.com/story/456953/

certified-health-coach-analee-joseph-helps-people-embark-on-their-journey-toward-body-transformation-with-optaviapowered-diet-plans.html

Roof Restoration | Roof Wash | Paint | Reseal. https://www.hawkesburyroofrestoration.com/roof-restoration/

Can Baby Sleep In Mamaroo Swing? (From Fussy To Peaceful). https://kidopick.com/can-baby-sleep-in-mamaroo-swing/

The Best Strategies to Increase Your Productivity - Citizen Coaching and Counselling Birmingham. https://citizencoaching.com/the-best-strategies-to-increase-your-productivity/

Three Tips To Reinvent Your Online Casino And Win – Casino Moon. https://casino-moon.com/three-tips-to-reinvent-your-online-casino-and-win/

Higher Order Functions | springerprofessional.de. https://www.springerprofessional.de/en/higher-order-functions/17050752

Which Has More Calories Beer or Wine? - Chill Beer. https://chillbeer.net/which-has-more-calories-beer-or-wine/

How to Lose Weight with Intermittent Fasting. https://best-today-good.com/how-to-lose-weight-with-intermittent-fasting/

Can You Drink Coffee While Intermittent Fasting?. https://eatforlonger.com/can-you-drink-coffee-while-intermittent-fasting/

Baskaran, K., Santhanam, S., & Ramakrishna, B. (2017). Association of ATG16L1 gene haplotype with inflammatory bowel disease in Indians. PLoS One, 12(5), e0178291.

Benefits of Intermittent fasting In Women's health - Blufashion. https://www.blufashion.com/lifestyle/health-wellness/benefits-of-intermittent-fasting-in-womens-health/

Wholesale Sign Up - Do-It-Yourself HCG. https://www.diyhcg.com/wholesale/wholesale-sign-up/

Healthy Eating 101: Simple Tips for Beginners to Transform Your Life! | littlecook. https://littlecook.io/blog/Healthy-Eating-101:-Simple-Tips-for-Beginners-to-Transform-Your-Life!

Lunch & Dinner Recipes Archives - Abbey's Kitchen. https://www.abbeyskitchen.com/category/recipes/lunch-dinner/

Caffeine Kick Start – Mama Megs. https://mamamegs.com/2017/02/03/caffeine-kick-start/

Mom & Toddler Simple Spinach Fruit Smoothie. https://www.themodelmentor.com/single-post/2018/08/08/mom-toddler-simple-spinach-fruit-smoothie

4 Beautiful Smoothie Bowls – TopTastyRecipes.com. https://www.toptastyrecipes.com/2022/08/10/4-beautiful-smoothie-bowls/

The BEST Easy Strawberry Smoothie Recipe Without Yogurt. https://24carrotkitchen.com/strawberry-smoothie/

Chicken Sausage Patties – 3010 Weight loss for life. https://3010weightlossforlife.com/recipes/chicken-sausage-patties/

Rachelâ€™s Favorite Quick & EASY Chicken Salad! | Clean Food Crush. https://cleanfoodcrush.com/quick-easy-chicken-salad-recipe/

How to make Creamy Cottage Cheese Crostini, recipe by MasterChef Sanjeev Kapoor. https://www.sanjeevkapoor.com/Recipe/Creamy-Cottage-Cheese-Crostini.html

5 Ways To Stick With Your Vegan Meal Plan in Raleigh NC. https://www.refectionfoods.com/post/5-ways-to-stick-with-your-vegan-meal-plan-in-raleigh-nc

banana | Davey Wavey Fitness. https://www.daveywaveyfitness.com/tag/banana/

Levo pa71:Trustworthy Review of 2023 - News Beyond Imagination. https://forbestimesonly.com/levo-pa71/

Beyond White Rice: Discovering the Nutritional Value of Whole Grains – Lilzone. https://lilzone.com/beyond-white-rice-discovering-the-nutritional-value-of-whole-grains/

PHYSALIS PROMAN FORTE 30 VTabs. https://justvegan.website/products/PHYSALIS-PROMAN-FORTE-30-VTabs-p366502993

Jack Beans Health Benefits - Barbell Rush. https://barbellrush.com/jack-beans-health-benefits/

7 Best Gluten-Free Plant-Based Protein Alternatives | blog, camping food, food and more | Nomad Nutrition What's Cookin'? blog. https://www.nomadnutrition.co/blogs/whats-cookin/gluten-free-plant-protein

Can Dogs Eat Sugar Snap Peas? - My Pet Experts. https://mypetexperts.com/can-dogs-eat-sugar-snap-peas/

Lemon Roasted Salmon | Produce For Kids. https://healthyfamilyproject.com/recipes/lemon-roasted-salmon/

6 Best Healthiest Foods for Kids [2022]. https://hiyahealth.com/blogs/news/healthy-food-for-kids

Plant-Based Intuitive Eating Wellness Blog – Morgan Bettini. https://morganbettini.com/category/blog/

Foods to Eat & Avoid During Pregnancy - The Wellness Mantra. https://www.thewellnessmantra.com/web-stories/foods-to-eat-avoid-during-pregnancy/

What are the disadvantages of tomato soup? – Need To Refrigerate. https://needtorefrigerate.com/what-are-the-disadvantages-of-tomato-soup/

10 Best Anti-Inflammatory Foods. https://www.martindalesnutrition.com/top-10-anti-inflammatory-foods/

Are Coffee & Tea Bad For You? - Gail Brady Nutrition. https://gailbradynutrition.com/are-coffee-tea-bad-for-you/

Are You Following These Recommended Physical Activity Guidelines? Bookmarkrocket. https://www.bookmarkrocket.com/story/are-you-following-these-recommended-physical-activity-guidelines/

Top 5 Tips for Elderly Dieting - A Nation of Moms. https://anationofmoms.com/2021/01/elderly-diets.html

What Are Antioxidants? (Here's What You Should Know). https://youeatplants.com/what-are-antioxidants/

Small but Mighty Micronutrients. https://www.lisaswifthealthyliving.com/post/small-but-mighty-micronutrients

Mellitox Reviews 2023 • Consumer Report • Is it a Scam?. https://www.dumblittleman.com/mellitox-reviews/

Discover the Amazing Health Benefits of Adding Seeds to Your Diet! | littlecook. https://littlecook.io/blog/Discover-the-Amazing-Health-Benefits-of-Adding-Seeds-to-Your-Diet!

Healthy Brunch Ideas - My Quick Recipes. https://myquickrecipes.com/healthy-brunch-ideas/

Berry High Fiber Starter – IsabellaMD. https://isabellamd.com/recipes/berry-high-fiber-starter/

Aéropostale Sunshine State Of Mind Flip-Top Water Bottle | Mall of America®. https://shop.mallofamerica.com/product/sunshine-state-of-mind-flip-top-water-bottle-aeropostale-f57f4d?model=0&variant=0

⬦ Glowing Skin, Naturally ⬦. https://www.annaviva.com/health/glowing-skin-naturally/

What Is The Difference In Gelato And Ice Cream?. https://kitsunerestaurant.com/what-is-the-difference-in-gelato-and-ice-cream/

What To Serve With Pesto Chicken? 12 Must-try Side Dishes - EpicureDelight. https://fooddc.org/pesto-chicken-sides/

Community | My Site. https://www.lokahicollective.com/community

Benefits of Leafy Greens for Skin. https://royaltyfastfood.com/benefits-of-leafy-greens/

bacteria – Reviews 2. https://reviews2.wpaffiliatemachine.com/tag/bacteria/

Blueberry – MTL Bagel Shop : Best hand rolled wood fire oven bagels in Montreal. https://mtlbagel.ca/product/blueberry/

Chickpea & Beet Veggie Burger | Earth Origins Market. https://earthoriginsmarket.com/lifestyle/recipes/chickpea-beet-veggie-burger

30-Minute Kid's Bagel Bite Lunch. https://tasty.co/recipe/easy-bagel-bite-lunch-ideas-for-kids

Shrimp Stuffed Salmon - Inspirational Momma. https://www.inspirationalmomma.com/shrimp-stuffed-salmon/

Dijon Pecan Salmon Recipe With Avocado Oil Mayonnaise – Hunter and Gather Foods. https://hunterandgatherfoods.com/blogs/recipes/dijon-pecan-salmon-recipe-with-avocado-oil-mayonnaise

Ryazhenka – baked & yogurted milk – ferment pittsburgh. https://fermentpittsburgh.com/2021/02/19/ryazhenka-baked-yogurted-milk/

Oolong Poached Peaches | Tea Pairing | JING Tea. https://jingtea.com/journal/oolong-poached-peaches-tea-and-food-pairing

GRIGLIATA MISTA DI CARNE ALL'ITALIANA. http://www.moletto.com/eng/recipes/italian_style_mixed_grill-85

Hey Sugar Sugar – GraceLaced. https://gracelaced.com/blogs/blog/hey-sugar-sugar

Best Weight Loss Breakfast Recipes » Top Tips To Reduce Weight In 2023. https://cure.care/best-weight-loss-breakfast-recipes/

Chilli Vegetarian. https://bosskitchen.com/chilli-vegetarian/

Barley Corn Salad. https://www.earthspirithearth.com/barley-corn-salad.html

A fit philosophy healthy gluten free easy recipes. https://cecorp.com/a-fit-philosophy-healthy-gluten-free-easy-recipes/

Food loss and waste in a changing environment — Research@WUR. https://research.wur.nl/en/publications/food-loss-and-waste-in-a-changing-environment

Wilkins Works inc - Zone 7 Schools' Program. https://www.wilkinsworksinc.com/zone-7-schools-program

Why are Children More Susceptible to Dehydration?. http://www.emergencymedicalparamedic.com/why-are-children-more-susceptible-to-dehydration/

How to Prevent the Appearance of Eye Wrinkles - Lavelier. https://www.lavelier.com/how-to-prevent-the-appearance-of-eye-wrinkles/

Local 871 News | How To Beat The Heat On Set. https://www.ialocal871.org/About-Us/Local-871-News/PostId/1418/how-to-beat-the-heat-on-set

The Ongoing Quest for Evidence on the Health Effects of Cannabis and Cannabis-Derived Products > Premier Research. https://premier-research.com/blog-cannabis-evidence-health/

Improve Digestion By Using This 12 Foods & Beverages. https://anaayafoods.com/improve-digestion/

Top 11 Fitness Attendant Certifications | ResumeCat. https://resumecat.com/blog/fitness-attendant-certifications

What is a Ketogenic Diet - A Complete Guide To Keto. https://ketokit.net/

Adaptogen Latte: Mushroom and Cacao Drink Recipe - Superfood Journal. https://superfoodjournal.com/mushroom-cacao-latte-drink/

Minted Peas Recipe - Feed Your Sole. https://feed-your-sole.com/minted-peas/

5 Simple Strategies to Stay Focused and Achieve Your Goals – Planndu Blog. https://planndu.com/blog/5-simple-strategies-to-stay-focused-and-achieve-your-goals/

Why Do I Feel So Tired Without Doing Anything? – From Doctor. https://fromdoctor.com/why-do-i-feel-so-tired-without-doing-anything.html

#affirmations | Flow Total Wellness. https://www.flowtotalwellness.com/tags/affirmations

Importance of Hydration. https://www.investassurellc.com/importance-of-hydration

Athletic Training and Therapy Ebook With HK Propel Access – Human Kinetics Canada. https://canada.humankinetics.com/products/athletic-training-and-therapy-ebook-with-hkpropel-access

Athletic Training and Therapy Ebook With HK Propel Access – Human Kinetics Canada. https://canada.humankinetics.com/products/athletic-training-and-therapy-ebook-with-hkpropel-access

7 Tips to Make Exercise a Daily Habit - Dr. Donald Waldrep. https://drwaldrep.com/blog/7-tips-to-make-exercise-a-daily-habit/

Healthy Eating Adds Up to a Healthy Heart - Better Vibrant Health. https://bettervibranthealth.com/healthy-heart/

Schreiber, M. (2019). Erectile Dysfunction. Medsurg Nursing, 28(5), 327.

Lectins In Canned Beans | How To Cure Diabetes Naturally. http://howtocurediabetesnaturally.net/lectins-in-canned-beans/

5 Tips for building a well rounded exercise plan | PMC Physiotherapy Dunboyne | Chartered Physiotherapists |. https://pmcphysiotherapy.ie/5-tips-for-building-a-well-rounded-exercise-plan/

Take the stairs - Direct Primary Care. https://www.dpcboca.com/take-the-stairs/

Personal | Needencouragement.com/personal-encouragement. https://needencouragement.com/personal-encouragement/

Exercise and Physical Activity: Benefits and Recommendations for a Healthy Lifestyle - En.ImArabic. https://en.imarabic.com/exercise-and-physical-activity-benefits-and-recommendations-for-a-healthy-lifestyle/

Ebix Blog | Webinar. https://blog.ebix.com/topic/webinar

5 disadvantages of drinking excessive tea. https://thepakistan.pk/5-disadvantages-of-drinking-excessive-tea/

Consider These Benefits of Exercise: Nova Physician Wellness Center: Weight Loss Specialists. https://www.novaphysicianwellness.com/blog/consider-these-benefits-of-exercise

Sleep Consultancy | Solutions Educational Psychology Ltd.. https://www.solutionseducationalpsychology.com/services-1

4 Excellent Ways To Improve The Quality Of Your Sleep – Allcityflooring. https://allcityfloorings.com/4-excellent-ways-to-improve-the-quality-of-your-sleep/

How To Lose Weight naturally - 37R. https://37r.net/how-to-lose-weight-naturally/

The Best Ways to Fall Asleep for Girls Who Are Just so Tired …. https://lifestyle.allwomenstalk.com/best-ways-to-fall-asleep/

Tips for a good night's sleep – Soul Performance Nutrition. https://www.soulperformancenutrition.com/blogs/news/tips-for-a-good-nights-sl

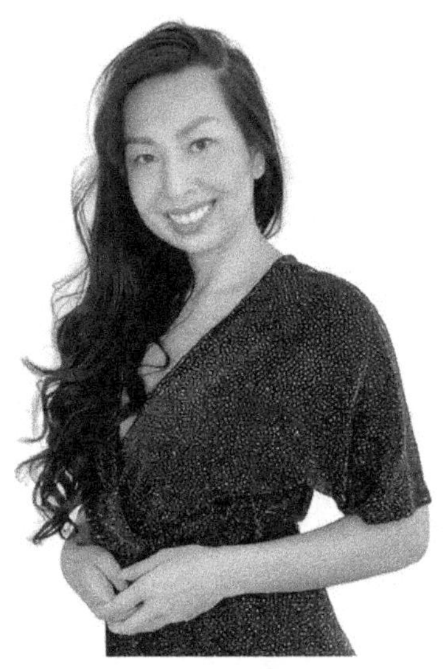

About the Author

Nancy Tran is a passionate advocate for holistic health and nutrition. With a deep-rooted belief in the transformative power of healthy living, she has dedicated her life to helping others achieve their wellness goals. Nancy is a Registered Holistic Nutritionist (RHN) and Certified Strength and Conditioning Specialist (CSS) with extensive knowledge and experience in the field.

Her compassionate approach and personalized guidance have empowered countless individuals to make positive life changes. Through her 1-on-1 consultations and writings, Nancy strives to simplify the complexities of healthy eating, making it accessible and enjoyable for everyone.

Nancy's expertise extends beyond nutrition as she recognizes the interconnectedness of mind, body, and soul. Her holistic approach emphasizes the importance of mental well-being, self-care practices, and mindful living. She firmly believes nourishing the body with wholesome food is a gateway to achieving harmony and vitality.

As an author, Nancy's writing style is engaging, practical, and filled with genuine care for her readers. Her words inspire and motivate, guiding individuals towards a healthier lifestyle and equipping them with the tools to sustain their journey.

When she's not immersed in the world of nutrition, Nancy enjoys exploring nature, travelling, experimenting with new recipes in the kitchen, and spending quality time with loved ones. Her genuine passion for health and wellness shines through in all aspects of her life, making her a trusted source of inspiration and knowledge.

Through this book and her various endeavours, Nancy seeks to empower individuals to take charge of their health, cultivate self-love, and embrace the transformative power of a healthy lifestyle.

Read more at https://www.holisticpharmacyandnutrition.com/.

9 798821 562474

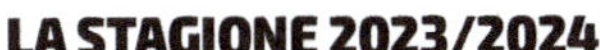

LA STAGIONE 2023/2024

	Avversario	Casa / Fuori	Risultato		Arbitro
			Vinta Nulla Persa		
PRIMA FASE					
1	**Napoli Femminile**	C	2-1	Vinta	Silvia Gasperotti
2	**Roma Femminile**	F	4-1	Persa	Gabriele Totaro
3	**Sampdoria Femminile**	F	1-2	Vinta	Edoardo M. Mazzoni
4	**Milan Femminile**	C	0-0	Nulla	Abdoulaye Diop
5	**Sassuolo Femminile**	F	1-2	Vinta	Andrea Zoppi
6	**Inter Women**	C	2-1	Vinta	Mattia Ubaldi
7	**Juventus Women**	C	0-3	Persa	Andrea Calzavara
8	**Fiorentina Femminile**	F	3-0	Persa	Fabrizio Pacella
9	**Pomigliano Femminile**	C	0-0	Nulla	Ermes F. Cavaliere
10	**Napoli Femminile**	F	0-0	Nulla	Simone Galipo
11	**Roma Femminile**	C	2-3	Persa	Mattia Nigro
12	**Sampdoria Femminile**	C	0-1	Persa	Enrico Cappai
13	**Milan Femminile**	F	3-2	Persa	Davide Gandino
14	**Sassuolo Femminile**	C	0-1	Persa	Edoardo M. Mazzoni
15	**Inter Women**	F	2-3	Vinta	Gioele Iacobellis
16	**Juventus Women**	F	5-0	Persa	Gianluca Catanzaro
17	**Fiorentina Femminile**	C	0-1	Persa	Alfredo Iannello
18	**Pomigliano Femminile**	F	3-4	Vinta	Valerio Pezzopane
POULE SALVEZZA					
1	**Napoli Femminile**	C	1-1	Nulla	Mattia Nigro
2	**Sampdoria Femminile**	F	1-0	Persa	Gabriele Restaldo
3	**Milan Femminile**	C	1-4	Persa	Lucio Felice Angelillo
4	**Pomigliano Femminile**	F	1-2	Vinta	Gabriele Restaldo
6	**Napoli Femminile**	F	1-1	Nulla	Emanuele Ceriello
7	**Sampdoria Femminile**	C	3-1	Vinta	Alberto Poli
8	**Milan Femminile**	F	1-0	Persa	Francesco Burlando
9	**Pomigliano Femminile**	C	2-0	Vinta	Gioele Iacobellis

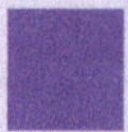

FIORENTINA FEMMINILE

ACF Fiorentina s.p.a.

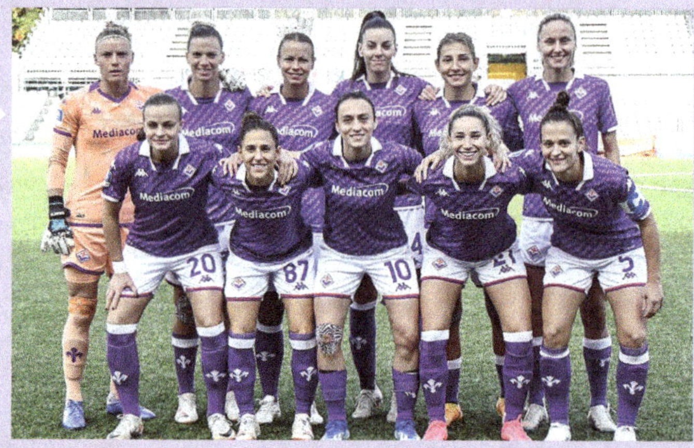

2015

Viola

Via Pian di Ripoli, 5 - 50012 Bagno a Ripoli (FI)

Curva Fiesole - Viola Park - Via Pian di Ripoli, 5 - 50012 Bagno a Ripoli (FI)

ORGANIGRAMMA
Presidente Rocco Commisso.
Direttore sportivo Simone Mazzoncini.
Responsabile calcio femminile Elena Turra.
Team manager Nicola Cecconi.

STAFF TECNICO
Allenatore Sebastian De La Fuente.
Allenatrice in seconda Priscilla Del Prete.
Preparatori atletici Alessandro Buccolini, Giovanni De Gennaro, Ettore Iacopetti.
Preparatore dei portieri Carmelo Roselli.
Match analyst Simone Saravo

PROFILO X
ACF_Womens

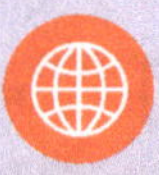

SITO INTERNET
acffiorentina.com

PAGINA FACEBOOK
acfwomens/

PROFILO INSTAGRAM
acf_women/

LA ROSA DELLA SQUADRA

Nome	Cognome	Nato il	PR	RE	AM	ES	SF	SA	Ruolo
Laura	**Agard**	26/07/1989	21	1	1	0	6	4	DIF
Rachele	**Baldi**	02/10/1994	13	0	1	0	0	0	POR
Melissa	**Bellucci**	08/02/2001	7	0	0	0	6	0	CEN
Veronica	**Boquete**	09/04/1987	24	9	1	0	1	7	CEN
Stephanie	**Breitner**	25/09/1992	10	0	1	0	3	5	CEN
Michela	**Catena**	17/12/1999	24	7	3	0	1	9	CEN
Norma	**Cinotti**	11/09/1996	13	1	1	0	8	5	CEN
Kaja	**Erzen**	21/08/1994	22	0	5	0	1	13	DIF
Emma	**Faerge**	06/12/2000	26	0	0	0	2	1	DIF
Marina	**Georgeva**	13/04/1997	22	0	3	1	2	3	DIF
Pauline	**Hammarlund**	07/05/1994	21	2	0	0	10	11	ATT
Madelena	**Janogy**	12/11/1995	14	7	0	0	4	7	CEN
Alexandra	**Johannsdottir**	19/03/2000	19	3	0	0	9	8	CEN
Zsanett Bernadet	**Kajan**	16/09/1997	6	2	0	0	3	3	ATT
Miriam	**Longo**	23/02/2000	24	4	3	0	12	11	ATT
Karin	**Lundin**	04/12/1994	15	1	0	0	8	6	ATT
Milica	**Mijatovic**	26/06/1991	22	2	2	0	9	12	CEN
Alice	**Parisi**	11/12/1990	19	0	3	0	13	6	CEN
Katja	**Schroffe- negger**	28/04/1991	13	0	3	0	0	0	POR
Emma	**Severini**	18/07/2003	25	0	6	0	1	9	CEN
Giorgia	**Spinelli**	12/12/1994	8	0	0	0	6	1	DIF
Martina	**Toniolo**	02/10/2001	22	0	5	0	14	5	DIF
Alice	**Tortelli**	22/01/1998	15	0	1	0	1	2	DIF
Linda	**Tucceri Cimini**	04/04/1991	7	0	0	0	6	0	DIF
Martina	**Zanoli**	27/02/2002	2	0	0	0	2	0	DIF

LEGENDA PR presenze - **RE** reti - **A** ammonizioni - **E** espulsioni - **SF** sostituzioni fatte - **SA** sostituzioni avute

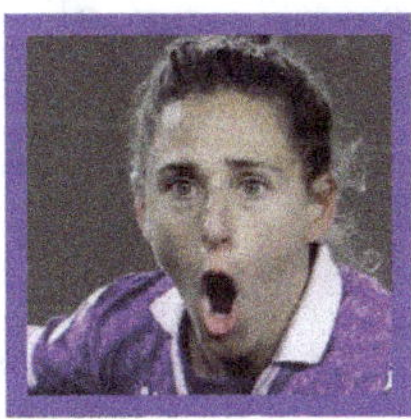

Veronica Boquete: Oltre a vincere la classifica degli assist (8) va a segno 9 volte

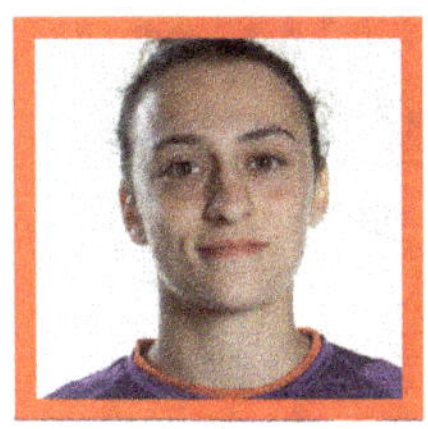

Michela Catena: Sette gol (suo personale in A) e 3 assist per la centrocampista viola

IL COMMENTO DELLA STAGIONE

Stagione da ricordare per la Fiorentina. La Viola si assicura dopo tre anni di assenza il ritorno nella Women's Champions League terminando il campionato al terzo posto. Obiettivo centrato grazie a una regular season di primissimo livello da parte della squadra di Sebastian De La Fuente: 12 vittorie a fronte di 3 sole sconfitte, maturate per altro contro le big del campionato. Dopo l'approdo alla finale di Coppa Italia la Fiorentina accusa nella Poule Scudetto un calo vistosissimo che non le preclude comunque la qualificazione continentale essendo riuscita a conservare sei dei tredici punti di vantaggio sul Sassuolo. Da sottolineare il rendimento offerto da Veronica Boquete e Michela Catena.

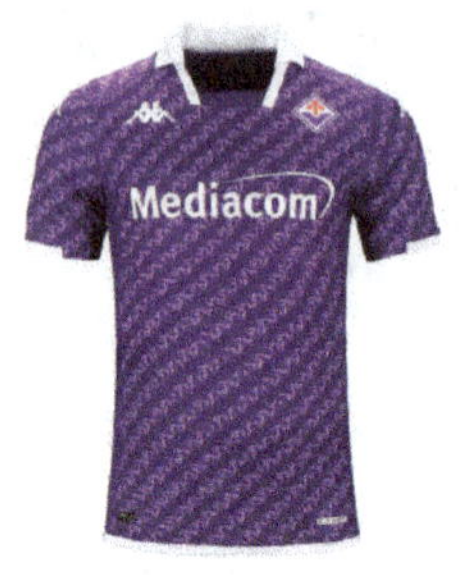
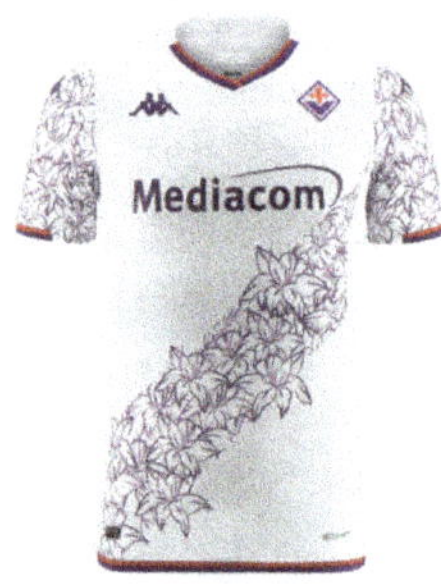
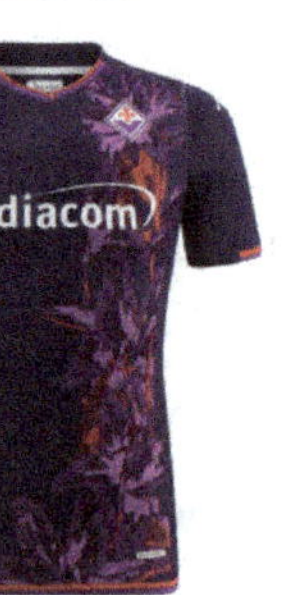

ANDAMENTO IN CAMPIONATO

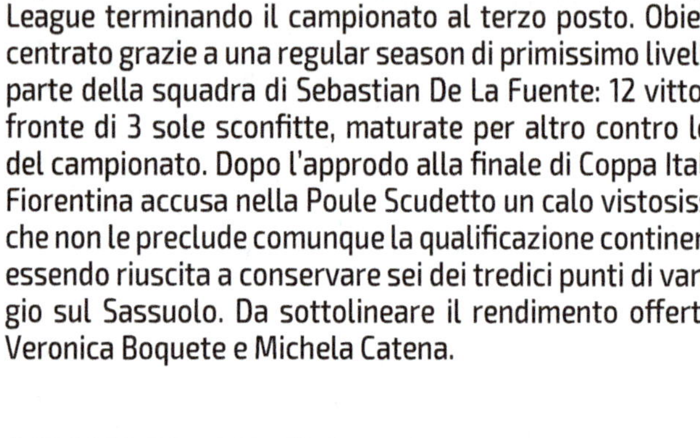

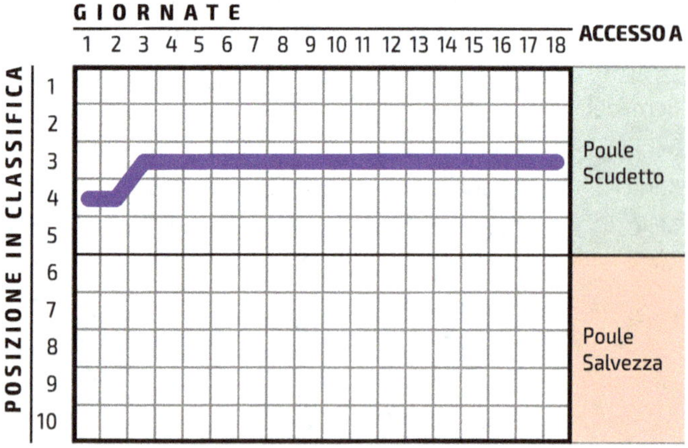

COMPORTAMENTO DELLA SQUADRA

Statistiche		Classifica										Rank
		10	09	08	07	06	05	04	03	02	01	
Giocatrici schierate	25											6
Giocatrici in rete	11											4
Giocatrici under 18	2											9
Giocatrici over 30	16											2
Cartellini gialli	28											6
Cartellini rossi	1											6
Cambi effettuati	90											1

LA STAGIONE 2023/2024

	Avversario	Casa / Fuori	Risultato	Arbitro
PRIMA FASE				
1	**Sassuolo Femminile**	C	2-1	Juan Luca Sacchi
2	**Inter Women**	F	1-1	Andrea Calzavara
3	**Napoli Femminile**	C	2-0	Luca Cherchi
4	**Pomigliano Femminile**	F	1-4	Dario Di Francesco
5	**Juventus Women**	C	1-2	Francesco Zago
6	**Milan Femminile**	C	1-0	Michele Delrio
7	**Sampdoria Femminile**	F	0-1	Maria Marotta
8	**Como Women**	C	3-0	Fabrizio Pacella
9	**Roma Femminile**	F	2-1	Silvia Gasperotti
10	**Sassuolo Femminile**	F	1-2	Gabriele Sacchi
11	**Inter Women**	C	4-2	Gabriele Scatena
12	**Napoli Femminile**	F	2-4	Erminio Cerbasi
13	**Pomigliano Femminile**	C	3-1	Simone Gavini
14	**Juventus Women**	F	2-2	Mattia Drigo
15	**Milan Femminile**	F	2-2	Edoardo Gianquinto
16	**Sampdoria Femminile**	C	2-1	Filippo Colaninno
17	**Como Women**	F	0-1	Alfredo Iannello
18	**Roma Femminile**	C	0-1	Giorgio Vergaro
POULE SCUDETTO				
1	**Sassuolo Femminile**	F	1-0	Alberto Poli
2	**Inter Women**	C	0-3	Andrea Calzavara
3	**Juventus Women**	F	4-0	Carlo Rinaldi
5	**Roma Femminile**	C	0-0	Carlo Rinaldi
6	**Sassuolo Femminile**	C	4-4	Antonio Di Reda
7	**Inter Women**	F	2-2	Stefano Milone
8	**Juventus Women**	C	0-2	Jules R. A. Tona Mbei
10	**Roma Femminile**	F	5-0	Valerio Vogliacco

INTER WOMEN
FC Internazionale Milano

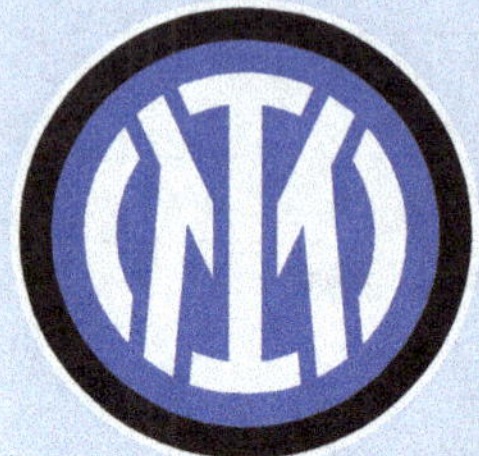

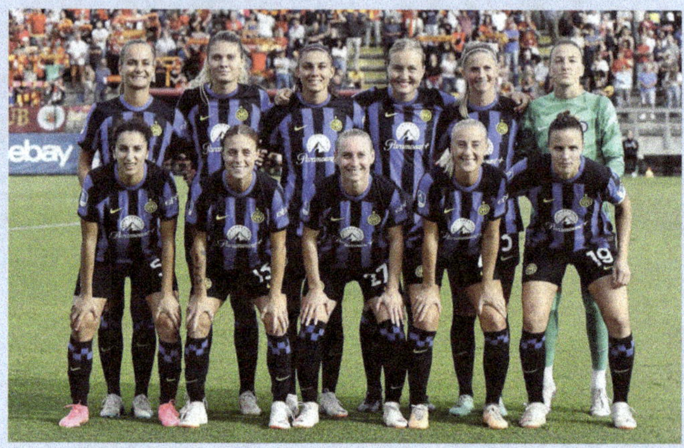

ANNO DI FONDAZIONE
2018

ORGANIGRAMMA
Presidente Zhang Kangyang.

COLORI SOCIALI
Nero Azzurro

STAFF TECNICO
Allenatrice Rita Guarino.
Allenatore in seconda Giorgio Schiavini.
Preparatori atletici Mario Familari, Andrea Bruno.
Preparatore dei portieri Gabriele Zanon.
Match analyst Alberto Angelastri

INDIRIZZO SEDE
Viale della
Liberazione, 16/18
- 20124 Milano

STADIO
**Arena Civica
Gianni Brera**
- Viale Giorgio
Byron, 2 - 20124
Milano

PROFILO X
Inter_Women/

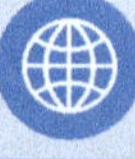
SITO INTERNET
inter.it

PAGINA FACEBOOK
Inter/

PROFILO INSTAGRAM
inter/

LA ROSA DELLA SQUADRA

Nome	Cognome	Nato il	PR	RE	AM	ES	SF	SA	Ruolo
Lisa	**Alborghetti**	19/06/1993	18	0	3	0	1	3	DIF
Tatiana	**Bonetti**	15/12/1991	11	0	0	0	10	1	ATT
Agnese	**Bonfantini**	04/07/1999	23	8	3	0	2	15	ATT
Katie	**Bowen**	15/04/1994	23	0	0	0	1	0	DIF
Haley	**Bugeja**	05/05/2004	22	4	0	0	10	11	ATT
Michela	**Cambiaghi**	04/02/1996	21	7	1	0	1	8	ATT
Sara	**Cetinja**	16/04/2000	23	0	0	0	1	0	POR
Henrietta	**Csiszar**	15/05/1994	23	1	4	0	4	15	CEN
Francesca	**Durante**	12/02/1997	4	0	0	0	0	1	POR
Noor	**Eckhoff**	06/12/1999	3	0	0	0	2	1	CEN
Beatrix	**Fordos**	07/01/2002	8	0	1	0	2	0	DIF
Maja	**Jelcic**	20/07/2004	15	1	0	0	15	0	ATT
Sofie	**Junge Pedersen**	24/04/1992	13	2	0	0	5	3	CEN
Ghoutia	**Karchouni**	29/05/1995	10	1	4	0	1	5	CEN
Lina	**Magull**	15/08/1994	14	9	1	0	1	3	CEN
Beatrice	**Merlo**	23/02/1999	11	0	0	0	2	2	DIF
Marija Ana	**Milinkovic**	16/11/2004	11	0	3	0	0	2	CEN
Ajara	**Nchout Njoya**	12/01/1993	5	0	0	0	4	1	ATT
Marta Teresa	**Pandini**	21/03/1998	12	0	0	0	7	3	CEN
Matilde	**Pavan**	12/06/2004	1	0	0	0	1	0	ATT
Elisa	**Polli**	27/08/2000	22	4	2	0	12	9	ATT
Chiara	**Robustellini**	30/06/2003	18	1	2	0	4	5	DIF
Anja	**Sonstevold**	21/06/1992	9	0	0	0	1	2	DIF
Irene	**Santi**	08/10/1999	5	0	0	0	3	1	CEN
Annamaria	**Serturini**	13/05/1998	7	4	0	0	1	4	ATT
Flaminia	**Simonetti**	17/02/1997	19	2	4	0	9	4	CEN
Frederikke Skjodt	**Thogersen**	24/07/1995	23	0	0	0	3	3	DIF
Andrine	**Tomter**	05/02/1995	18	0	0	0	3	4	DIF

LEGENDA PR presenze - **RE** reti - **A** ammonizioni - **E** espulsioni - **SF** sostituzioni fatte - **SA** sostituzioni avute

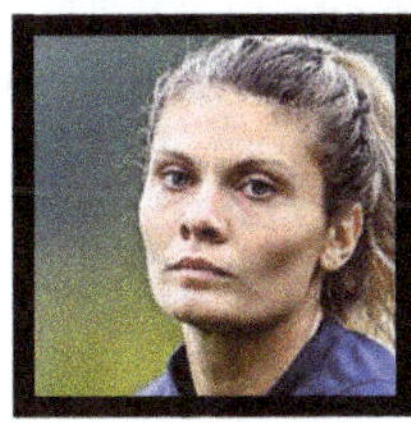

Michela Cambiaghi: Sette gol e 4 assist nella prima stagione all'Inter per l'azzurra

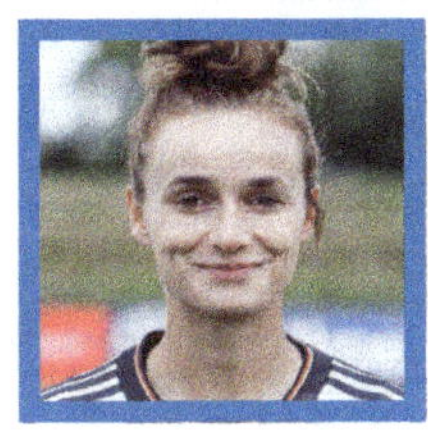

Lina Magul: L'ex Bayern Monaco si rivela la miglior realizzatrice nerazzurra (9 gol)

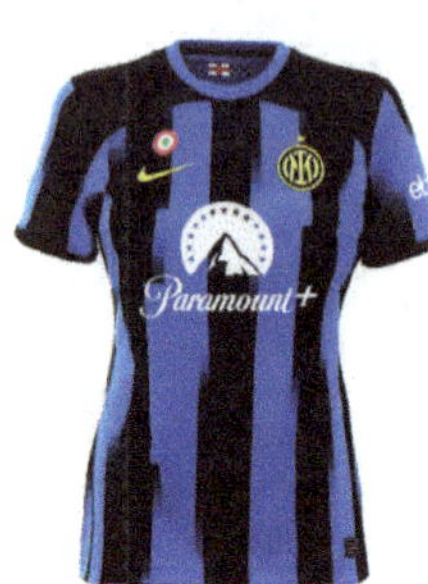

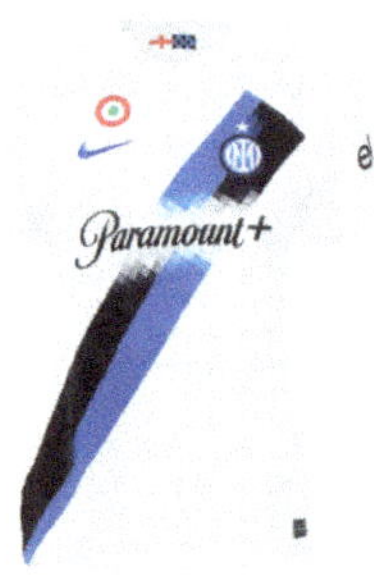

IL COMMENTO DELLA STAGIONE

L'Inter termina il campionato in quinta posizione per la terza volta di fila. Le nerazzurre, nel girone di ritorno della regular season, non riescono a conservare il quarto posto con il quale avevano virato al giro di boa. La Poule Scudetto lascia l'amaro in bocca all'Inter. La formazione di Rita Guarino si fa apprezzare in trasferta andando a cogliere brillanti affermazioni contro Juventus e Fiorentina. A rendere irrealizzabile un tentativo di rimonta in chiave europea è il rendimento offerto all'Arena Civica (due miseri punti in quattro gare). Tra le note positive della stagione sono da segnalare la centrocampista tedesca Lina Magull e le attaccanti Agnese Bonfantini e Michela Cambiaghi.

ANDAMENTO IN CAMPIONATO

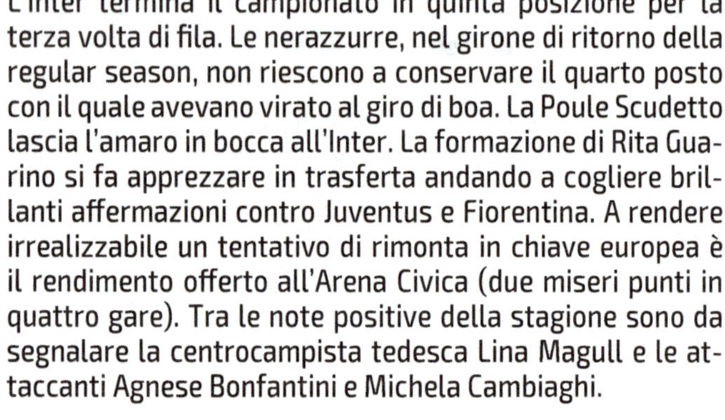

COMPORTAMENTO DELLA SQUADRA

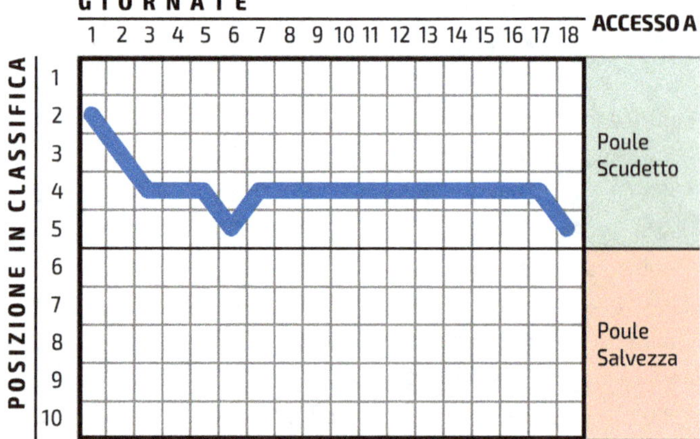

Statistiche		Classifica										Rank
		10	09	08	07	06	05	04	03	02	01	
Giocatrici schierate	28											1
Giocatrici in rete	12											3
Giocatrici under 18	9											1
Giocatrici over 30	6											9
Cartellini gialli	18											2
Cartellini rossi	0											1
Cambi effettuati	70											7

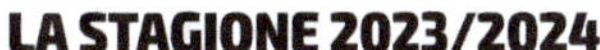

LA STAGIONE 2023/2024

	Avversario	Casa / Fuori	Risultato		Arbitro
PRIMA FASE					
1	**Sampdoria Femminile**	F	0-2	Vinta	Edoardo Gianquinto
2	**Fiorentina Femminile**	C	1-1	Nulla	Andrea Calzavara
3	**Sassuolo Femminile**	F	1-2	Vinta	Simone Galipo
4	**Roma Femminile**	F	2-0	Persa	Marco Emmanuele
5	**Napoli Femminile**	C	2-0	Vinta	Antonino Costanza
6	**Como Women**	F	2-1	Persa	Mattia Ubaldi
7	**Pomigliano Femminile**	C	2-1	Vinta	Stefano Nicolini
8	**Juventus Women**	F	5-0	Persa	L. Mastrodomenico
9	**Milan Femminile**	C	1-0	Vinta	Maria Marotta
10	**Sampdoria Femminile**	C	1-1	Nulla	Aleksandar Djurdjevic
11	**Fiorentina Femminile**	F	4-2	Persa	Gabriele Scatena
12	**Sassuolo Femminile**	C	0-1	Persa	Marco Peletti
13	**Roma Femminile**	C	2-0	Vinta	Samuele Andreano
14	**Napoli Femminile**	F	2-3	Vinta	Gabriele Sacchi
15	**Como Women**	C	2-3	Persa	Gioele Iacobellis
16	**Pomigliano Femminile**	F	2-6	Vinta	Mario Perri
17	**Juventus Women**	C	0-2	Persa	Maria Marotta
18	**Milan Femminile**	F	2-1	Persa	Matteo Centi
POULE SCUDETTO					
1	**Juventus Women**	C	3-3	Nulla	Andrea Ancora
2	**Fiorentina Femminile**	F	3-3	Vinta	Andrea Calzavara
3	**Roma Femminile**	C	1-2	Persa	Andrea Zanotti
4	**Sassuolo Femminile**	F	2-1	Persa	Alessandro Silvestri
6	**Juventus Women**	F	0-2	Vinta	Gabriele Sacchi
7	**Fiorentina Femminile**	C	2-2	Nulla	Stefano Milone
8	**Roma Femminile**	F	4-3	Persa	Giuseppe Maria Manzo
9	**Sassuolo Femminile**	C	2-4	Persa	Francesco D'Eusanio

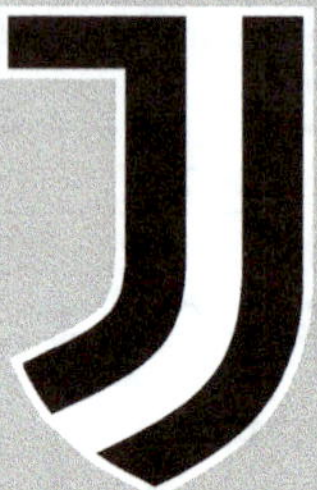

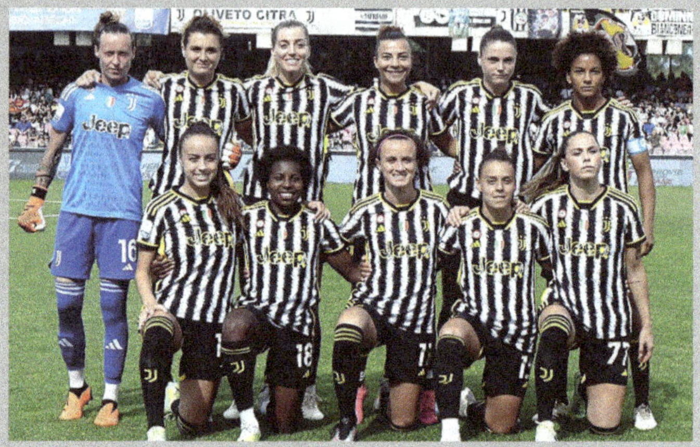

ANNO DI FONDAZIONE
2017

COLORI SOCIALI
Bianco Nero

INDIRIZZO SEDE
Via Druento, 175 -
10151 Torino

STADIO
Vittorio Pozzo
- La Marmora -
Viale Macallè, 21
- 13900 Biella

ORGANIGRAMMA
Presidente Gianluca Ferrero.
Head of women Stefano Braghin.
Team manager Raffaela Masciandri.

STAFF TECNICO
Allenatore Joe Montemurro (1-18), Giuseppe Zappella.
Preparatori atletici Emanuele Chiappero, Enrico Picco.
Preparatore dei portieri Giuseppe Mammoliti.
Match analyst Maeva Ruiz

PROFILO X
juventusfc/

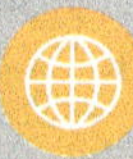

SITO INTERNET
juventus.com

PAGINA FACEBOOK
Juventus/

PROFILO INSTAGRAM
juventuswomen/

LA ROSA DELLA SQUADRA

Nome	Cognome	Nato il	PR	RE	AM	ES	SF	SA	Ruolo
Roberta	**Aprile**	22/11/2000	3	0	0	0	0	0	POR
Lineth	**Beerensteyn**	11/10/1996	23	7	0	0	4	7	ATT
Melissa	**Bellucci**	08/02/2001	4	0	1	0	4	0	CEN
Lisa	**Boattin**	03/05/1997	23	2	1	0	1	3	DIF
Barbara	**Bonansea**	13/06/1991	19	3	5	1	10	8	ATT
Asia	**Bragonzi**	05/03/2001	7	0	1	0	5	2	ATT
Federica	**Cafferata**	07/05/2000	5	0	0	0	3	2	CEN
Viola	**Calligaris**	17/03/1996	11	0	0	0	0	2	DIF
Sofia	**Cantore**	30/09/1999	20	4	0	0	4	14	ATT
Arianna	**Caruso**	06/11/1999	25	7	4	0	2	8	CEN
Estelle	**Cascarino**	05/02/1997	23	0	2	0	2	1	DIF
Jennifer	**Echegini**	22/03/2001	14	10	0	0	6	7	CEN
Sara	**Gama**	27/03/1989	16	0	1	0	11	3	DIF
Maelle	**Garbino**	09/08/1996	20	3	3	0	8	9	ATT
Cristiana	**Girelli**	23/04/1990	22	11	0	0	7	12	ATT
Julia Angela	**Grosso**	29/08/2000	21	6	1	0	1	6	CEN
Sara Bjork	**Gunnarsdottir**	29/09/1990	17	1	3	1	5	4	CEN
Martina	**Lenzini**	23/07/1998	24	0	3	0	2	10	DIF
Amanda	**Nilden**	07/08/1998	9	1	1	0	4	1	DIF
Paulina	**Nystrom**	17/08/2000	13	1	1	0	7	4	ATT
Ella	**Palis**	24/03/1999	11	0	0	0	8	2	CEN
Elsa Helena	**Pelgander**	02/08/2006	3	0	0	0	2	0	CEN
Pauline	**Peyraud-Magnin**	17/03/1992	23	0	5	0	0	0	POR
Cecilia	**Salvai**	02/12/1993	17	1	1	0	2	3	DIF
Linda	**Sembrant**	15/05/1987	2	0	0	0	1	0	DIF
Gloria	**Sliskovic**	04/05/2005	1	0	0	0	1	0	DIF
Lindsey Kimberly	**Thomas**	27/04/1995	23	8	0	0	13	5	ATT

LEGENDA PR presenze - **RE** reti - **A** ammonizioni - **E** espulsioni - **SF** sostituzioni fatte - **SA** sostituzioni avute

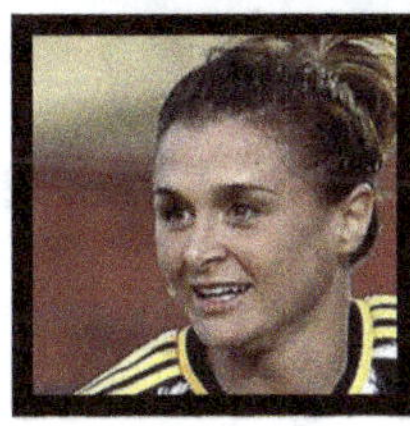

Cristiana Girelli: Terza miglior marcatrice del torneo alle spalle di Viens e Giacinti

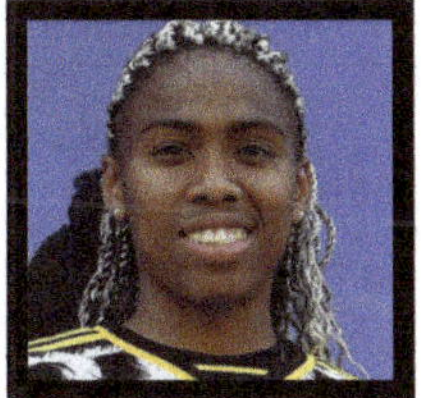

Lindsey Thomas: Otto gol e 4 assist alla 1ª stagione in bianconero per l'avanti francese

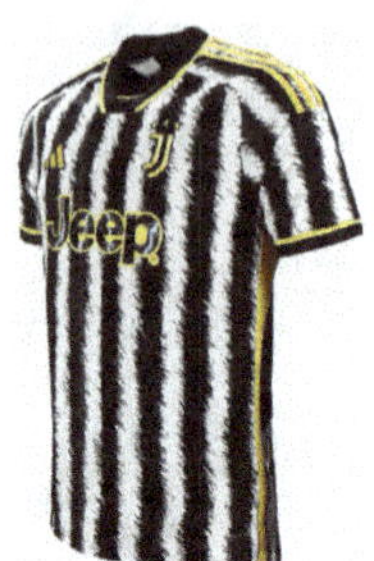

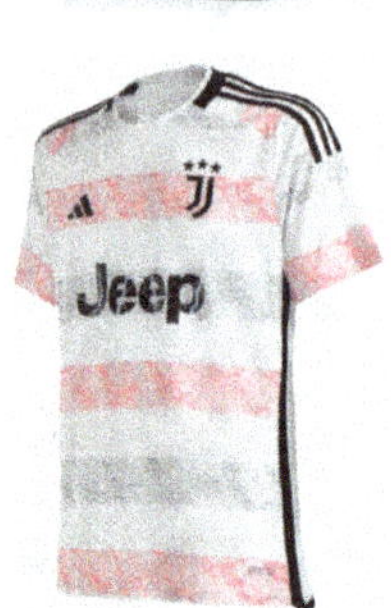

IL COMMENTO DELLA STAGIONE

Per la seconda stagione consecutiva la Juventus si deve accontentare della piazza d'onore. Le bianconere riescono a tenere il passo della Roma soltanto nella prima parte del campionato. Nel girone di ritorno il pareggio interno contro la Fiorentina e la sconfitta nel confronto diretto con le giallorosse allontanano la compagine torinese dalla prima della classe. A spegnere definitivamente le speranze di risalita della squadra di Giuseppe Zappella (subentrato a Joe Montemurro) nella Poule Scudetto sono i ko rimediati contro Inter e Roma. A livello individuale spiccano le prestazioni offerte dalla centrocampista Julia Grosso e dalle avanti Lineth Beerensteyn, Lindsey Thomas e Cristiana Girelli.

ANDAMENTO IN CAMPIONATO

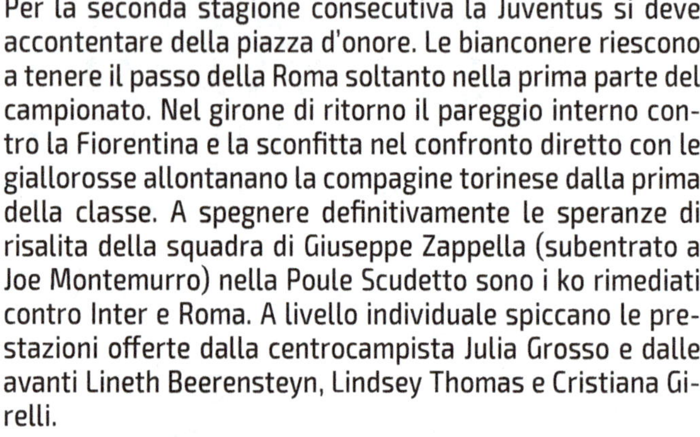

COMPORTAMENTO DELLA SQUADRA

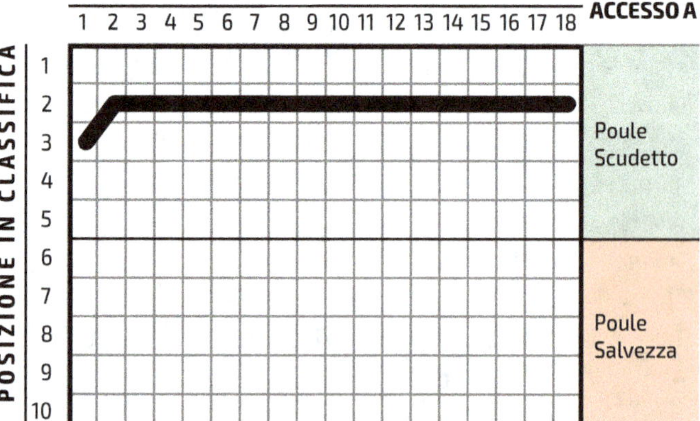

Statistiche		Classifica										Rank
		10	09	08	07	06	05	04	03	02	01	
Giocatrici schierate	26											3
Giocatrici in rete	13											1
Giocatrici under 18	7											2
Giocatrici over 30	11											3
Cartellini gialli	20											4
Cartellini rossi	1											6
Cambi effettuati	75											6

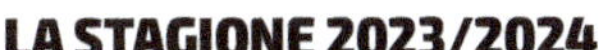

LA STAGIONE 2023/2024

	Avversario	Casa / Fuori	Risultato		Arbitro
			Vinta Nulla Persa		
PRIMA FASE					
1	**Pomigliano Femminile**	F	2-3	Vinta	Gabriele Totaro
2	**Sampdoria Femminile**	C	4-1	Vinta	Luca De Angeli
3	**Milan Femminile**	F	0-1	Vinta	Alberto Ruben Arena
4	**Sassuolo Femminile**	C	4-0	Vinta	Giuseppe Vingo
5	**Fiorentina Femminile**	F	1-2	Vinta	Francesco Zago
6	**Roma Femminile**	C	1-3	Persa	Domenico Mirabella
7	**Como Women**	F	0-3	Vinta	Andrea Calzavara
8	**Inter Women**	C	5-0	Vinta	L. Mastrodomenico
9	**Napoli Femminile**	F	1-3	Vinta	Samuele Andreano
10	**Pomigliano Femminile**	C	4-0	Vinta	Mattia Caldera
11	**Sampdoria Femminile**	F	1-0	Persa	Giorgio Bozzetto
12	**Milan Femminile**	C	2-1	Vinta	Lorenzo Maccarini
13	**Sassuolo Femminile**	F	0-1	Vinta	Andrea Ancora
14	**Fiorentina Femminile**	C	2-2	Nulla	Mattia Drigo
15	**Roma Femminile**	F	3-1	Persa	Marco Emmanuele
16	**Como Women**	C	5-0	Vinta	Gianluca Catanzaro
17	**Inter Women**	F	0-2	Vinta	Maria Marotta
18	**Napoli Femminile**	C	4-1	Vinta	Giorgio Bozzetto
POULE SCUDETTO					
1	**Inter Women**	F	3-3	Nulla	Andrea Ancora
3	**Fiorentina Femminile**	C	4-0	Vinta	Carlo Rinaldi
4	**Roma Femminile**	F	2-1	Persa	Lorenzo Maccarini
5	**Sassuolo Femminile**	C	2-1	Vinta	Gianluca Renzi
6	**Inter Women**	C	0-2	Persa	Gabriele Sacchi
8	**Fiorentina Femminile**	F	0-2	Vinta	Jules R. A. Tona Mbei
9	**Roma Femminile**	C	3-1	Vinta	Cristiano Ursini
10	**Sassuolo Femminile**	F	2-3	Vinta	Simone Gavini

AC Milan s.p.a.

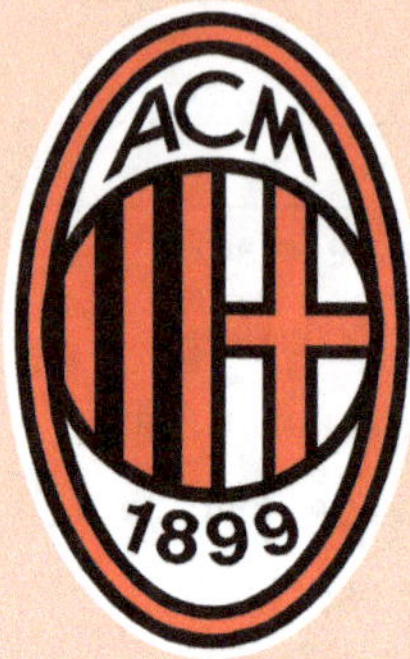

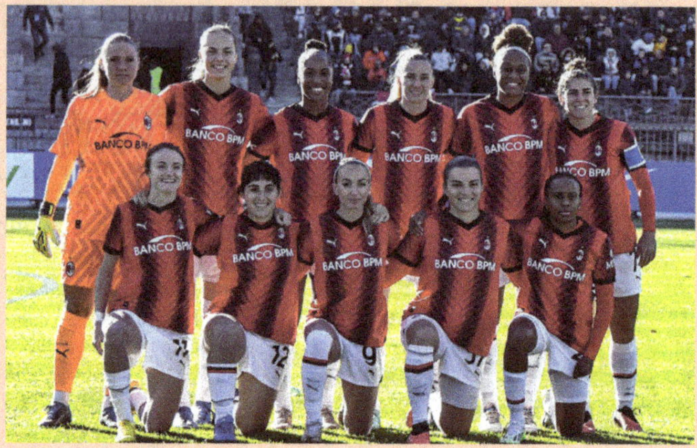

ANNO DI FONDAZIONE
2018

COLORI SOCIALI
Rosso Nero

INDIRIZZO SEDE
Via Aldo Rossi, 8 - 20149 Milano

STADIO
Puma House of Football - Centro Peppino Vismara - Via dei Missaglia, 117 - 20142 Milano

ORGANIGRAMMA
Presidente Paolo Scaroni.
Head of women Elisabet Spina.
Team manager Roberto Angioni.

STAFF TECNICO
Allenatore Maurizio Ganz (1-8), Davide Corti.
Allenatore in seconda Davide Cordone.
Preparatori atletici Matteo Callini.
Preparatore dei portieri Christian Berretta.
Match analyst Laura Brambilla

PROFILO X
acmilan/

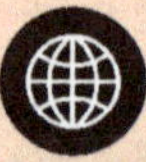

SITO INTERNET
acmilan.com

PAGINA FACEBOOK
ACMilan/

PROFILO INSTAGRAM
acmilan/

LA ROSA DELLA SQUADRA

Nome	Cognome	Nato il	PR	RE	AM	ES	SF	SA	Ruolo
Greta	**Adami**	30/07/1992	8	0	1	0	7	1	CEN
Gudny	**Arnadottir**	04/08/2000	10	0	0	0	4	2	DIF
Giorgia	**Arrigoni**	04/10/2004	2	0	0	0	2	0	ATT
Kosovare	**Asllani**	29/07/1989	17	6	1	0	4	8	ATT
Serena Delia	**Babb**	26/08/1995	5	0	1	0	0	1	POR
Valentina	**Bergamaschi**	22/01/1997	23	2	6	0	0	6	DIF
Valentina	**Cernoia**	22/06/1991	16	0	2	0	2	7	CEN
Matilde	**Copetti**	15/09/1997	1	0	0	0	1	0	POR
Chante M. D.	**Dompig**	12/02/2001	26	6	1	0	7	11	ATT
Kamila	**Dubcova**	17/01/1999	17	3	0	0	3	6	CEN
Laura	**Fusetti**	08/10/1990	8	0	0	0	5	1	DIF
Laura	**Giuliani**	05/06/1993	21	0	0	0	0	0	POR
Christy Louise	**Grimshaw**	08/11/1995	20	1	3	0	0	10	CEN
Alia	**Guagni**	01/10/1987	22	0	0	0	6	9	DIF
Evelin	**Ijeh**	12/08/2001	12	3	1	0	5	5	ATT
Rimante	**Jonusaite**	25/10/2003	1	0	0	0	1	0	ATT
Emelyne Ann-Emmanuelle	**Laurent**	04/11/1998	20	4	1	1	7	8	ATT
Gloria	**Marinelli**	12/03/1998	21	2	1	0	16	5	ATT
Marta	**Mascarello**	15/10/1998	20	2	5	0	6	11	CEN
Malgorzata G.	**Mesjasz**	12/06/1997	12	2	3	0	2	0	DIF
Nadia	**Nadim**	02/01/1988	8	0	0	0	3	5	ATT
Julie	**Piga**	12/01/1998	22	0	4	0	1	4	DIF
Silvia	**Rubio Avila**	12/10/2000	13	1	0	0	8	4	CEN
Angelica	**Soffia**	02/07/2000	16	1	1	0	9	2	DIF
Andrea	**Staskova**	12/05/2000	21	6	0	0	4	8	ATT
Allison	**Swaby**	03/10/1996	19	0	0	0	2	1	DIF
Sara	**Thrige Andersen**	15/05/1996	4	0	0	0	1	3	DIF
Valery	**Vigilucci**	15/04/1997	20	2	2	0	13	1	CEN
Sandro	**Tonali**	08/05/2000	34	2	9	0	4	7	CEN
Aster	**Vranckx**	04/09/2002	9	0	1	0	7	1	CEN

LEGENDA PR presenze - **RE** reti - **A** ammonizioni - **E** espulsioni - **SF** sostituzioni fatte - **SA** sostituzioni avute

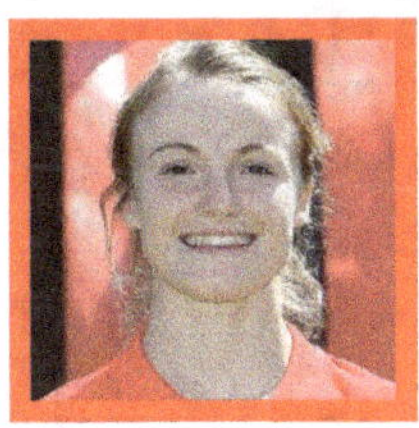

Christy Grimshaw: Una rete e 4 assist per la centrocampista scozzese del Milan

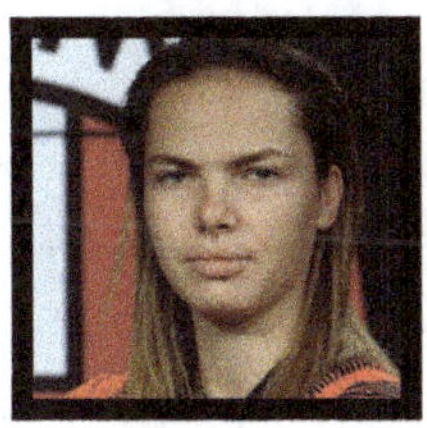

Andrea Staskova: Miglior realizzatrice rossonera (6 gol) insieme ad Asllani e Dompig

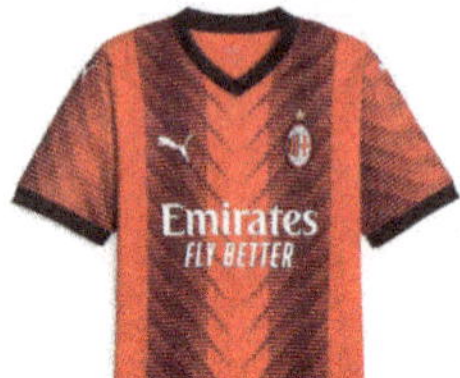

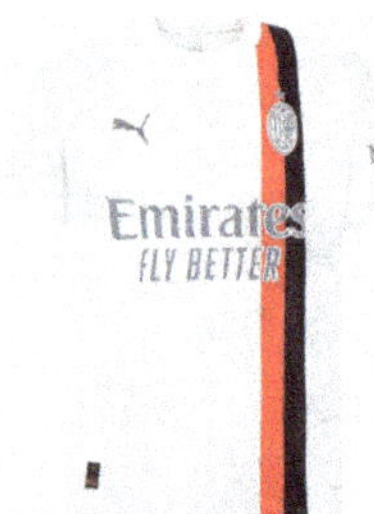

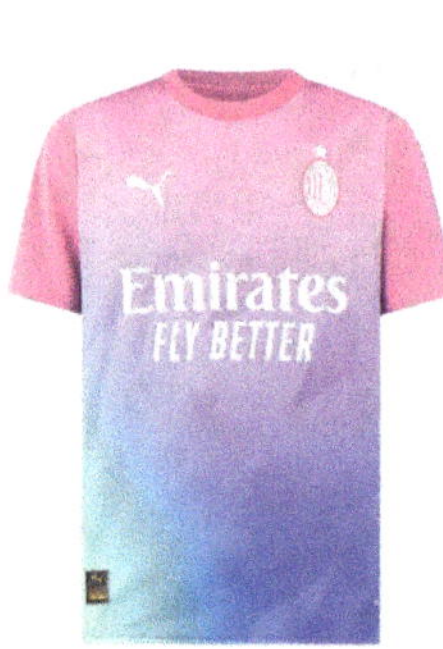

IL COMMENTO DELLA STAGIONE

Torneo in chiaroscuro per il Milan terminato al sesto posto. La partenza è a rilento. A pagare è il tecnico Maurizio Ganz esonerato dopo aver racimolato 9 punti in 8 gare. L'avvento in panchina di Davide Corti non sembra inizialmente dare frutti (1 punto in 4 incontri). La situazione migliora sensibilmente nell'ultimo terzo del girone di ritorno dove la squadra consegue 11 punti che gli consentono di finire la regular season al 6° posto. Nella Poule Salvezza ne giungono altri 20 che garantiscono al Milan la permanenza in A con largo anticipo, ma al tempo stesso lasciano il rammarico per una prima parte di stagione deludente. Bene le avanti Kosovare Asllani, Chante Dompig e Andrea Staskova.

ANDAMENTO IN CAMPIONATO

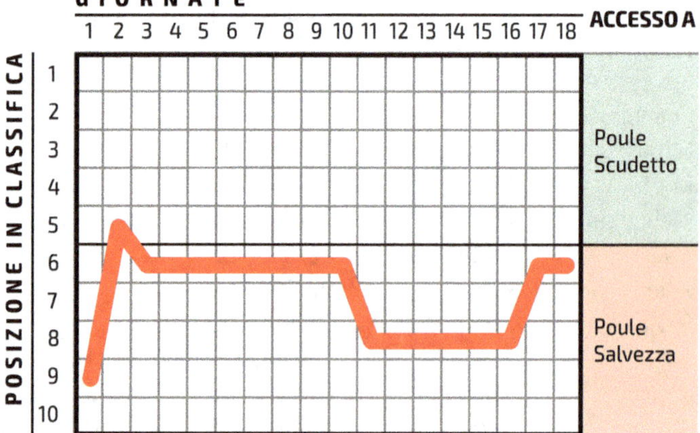

COMPORTAMENTO DELLA SQUADRA

Statistiche		Classifica										Rank
		10	09	08	07	06	05	04	03	02	01	
Giocatrici schierate	26											3
Giocatrici in rete	10											5
Giocatrici under 18	3											7
Giocatrici over 30	10											4
Cartellini gialli	27											5
Cartellini rossi	0											1
Cambi effettuati	80											3

LA STAGIONE 2023/2024

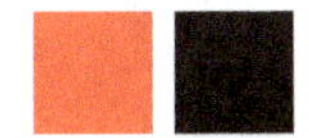

	Avversario	Casa / Fuori	Risultato		Arbitro
PRIMA FASE					
1	**Roma Femminile**	C	2-4	🟥	Domenico Castellone
2	**Napoli Femminile**	F	0-1	🟩	Mauro Gangi
3	**Juventus Women**	C	0-1	🟥	Alberto Ruben Arena
4	**Como Women**	F	0-0	⬜	Abdoulaye Diop
5	**Pomigliano Femminile**	C	4-1	🟩	Gabriele Sacchi
6	**Fiorentina Femminile**	F	1-0	🟥	Michele Delrio
7	**Sassuolo Femminile**	C	1-1	⬜	Carlo Rinaldi
8	**Sampdoria Femminile**	C	1-1	⬜	Giuseppe C. Allegretta
9	**Inter Women**	F	1-0	🟥	Maria Marotta
10	**Roma Femminile**	F	2-1	🟥	Filippo Giaccaglia
11	**Napoli Femminile**	C	1-1	⬜	Giuseppe Maria Manzo
12	**Juventus Women**	F	2-1	🟥	Lorenzo Maccarini
13	**Como Women**	C	3-2	🟩	Davide Gandino
14	**Pomigliano Femminile**	F	0-0	⬜	Domenico Leone
15	**Fiorentina Femminile**	C	2-2	⬜	Edoardo Gianquinto
16	**Sassuolo Femminile**	F	1-0	🟥	Eugenio Scarpa
17	**Sampdoria Femminile**	F	1-3	🟩	Simone Gauzolino
18	**Inter Women**	C	2-1	🟩	Matteo Centi
POULE SALVEZZA					
2	**Pomigliano Femminile**	C	4-0	🟩	Jules R. A. Tona Mbei
3	**Como Women**	F	1-4	🟩	Lucio Felice Angelillo
4	**Napoli Femminile**	C	3-2	🟩	Gabriele Totaro
5	**Sampdoria Femminile**	F	1-3	🟩	Edoardo M. Mazzoni
7	**Pomigliano Femminile**	F	2-2	⬜	Adolfo Baratta
8	**Como Women**	C	1-0	🟩	Francesco Burlando
9	**Napoli Femminile**	F	1-1	⬜	Giorgio Di Cicco
10	**Sampdoria Femminile**	C	3-1	🟩	Davide Gandino

Legenda risultato: 🟩 Vinta ⬜ Nulla 🟥 Persa

NAPOLI FEMMINILE

SSD ARL Napoli Femminile

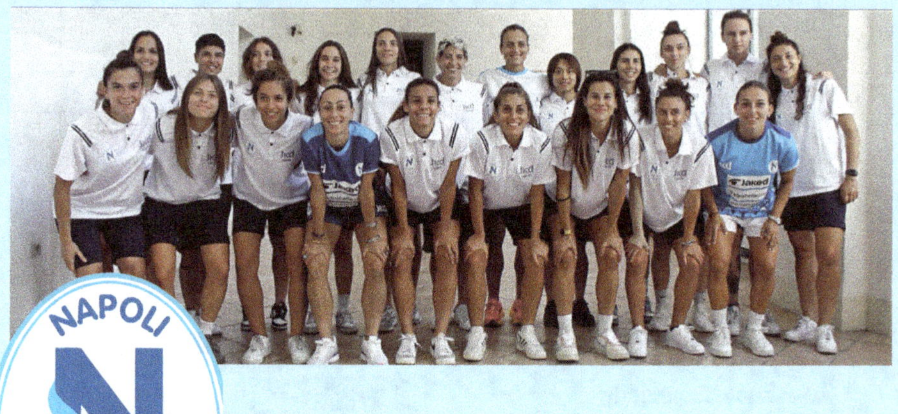

ANNO DI FONDAZIONE
2003 (2005)

COLORI SOCIALI
Azzurro

INDIRIZZO SEDE
Piazza dei Martiri,
30 - 80121 Napoli

ORGANIGRAMMA
Presidente Alessandro Maiello.
Direttore generale Marco Zwingauer.
Team manager Alessandra Nencioni.

STAFF TECNICO
Allenatore Biagio Seno.
Allenatore in seconda Andrea Marigliano.
Collaboratori tecnici Paolino Baldari.
Preparatori atletici Pasquale Perna.
Preparatore dei portieri Andrea Cerboneschi.
Fitness coach Michele Gristina

STADIO
Giuseppe Piccolo -Via Matilde Serao, 1 - 80040 Cercola
(NA)

PROFILO X
NapoliFemminile/

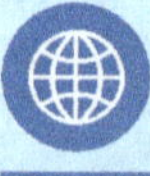

SITO INTERNET
napolifemminile.it

PAGINA FACEBOOK
ssdnapoli
femminile/

PROFILO INSTAGRAM
napolifemminile/

LA ROSA DELLA SQUADRA

Nome	Cognome	Nato il	PR	RE	AM	ES	SF	SA	Ruolo
Doris	**Bacic**	23/02/1995	20	0	3	0	0	0	POR
Marija	**Banusic eredinho**	17/09/1995	20	3	3	1	7	5	ATT
Beatrice	**Beretta**	01/07/2003	5	0	0	0	0	0	POR
Sofia	**Bertucci**	30/07/2004	20	0	1	0	10	6	DIF
Sara	**Cammarano**	06/01/2006	1	0	0	0	1	0	DIF
Gina Maria	**Chmielinski**	07/06/2000	25	1	3	0	2	9	CEN
Alice	**Corelli**	28/11/2003	23	2	4	0	15	6	ATT
Alessia	**D'Angelo**	25/05/2006	1	0	0	0	1	0	CEN
Elisa Mateu	**Del Estal**	23/03/1993	24	6	2	0	5	5	ATT
Martina	**Di Bari**	05/06/2002	19	0	6	0	5	5	DIF
Paola	**Di Marino**	04/05/1994	20	1	3	0	0	3	DIF
Francesca	**Fabiano**	15/04/2003	1	0	0	0	0	0	POR
Valentina	**Gallazzi**	16/07/2003	25	1	4	0	2	3	CEN
Giulia	**Giacobbo**	30/05/2003	22	1	2	0	9	12	CEN
Alice	**Giai**	09/01/2003	14	0	3	0	2	11	CEN
Morena	**Gianfico**	01/01/2008	6	0	1	0	6	0	ATT
Susanne	**Joy Friedichs**	29/10/1988	9	0	1	0	3	6	DIF
Nina	**Kajzba**	04/04/2004	15	0	1	0	11	3	CEN
Miharu	**Kobayashi**	12/10/1992	24	1	1	0	1	0	DIF
Gabriella	**Langella**	11/04/2007	1	0	0	0	1	0	CEN
Paloma	**Lazaro Torres Del Molino**	28/09/1993	23	2	5	0	8	11	ATT
Claudia	**Mauri**	18/12/1992	19	0	1	0	6	6	CEN
Alice	**Pellinghelli**	17/06/2003	17	0	0	0	1	7	DIF
Tecla	**Pettenuzzo**	30/11/1999	24	0	4	0	2	2	DIF
Yuki	**Togawa**	13/09/2000	1	0	0	0	0	0	CEN
Federica	**Veritti**	06/07/1999	7	0	2	0	2	0	DIF

LEGENDA PR presenze - **RE** reti - **A** ammonizioni - **E** espulsioni - **SF** sostituzioni fatte - **SA** sostituzioni avute

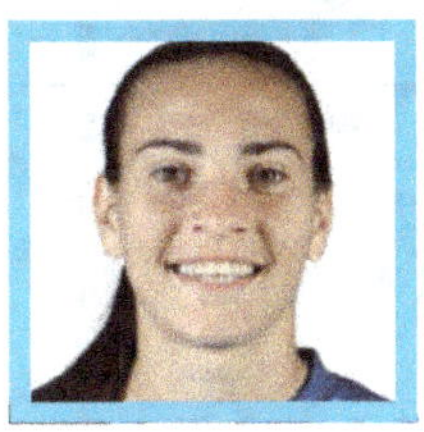

Alice Corelli: La giovane avanti chiude la sua prima stagione al Napoli con 2 reti

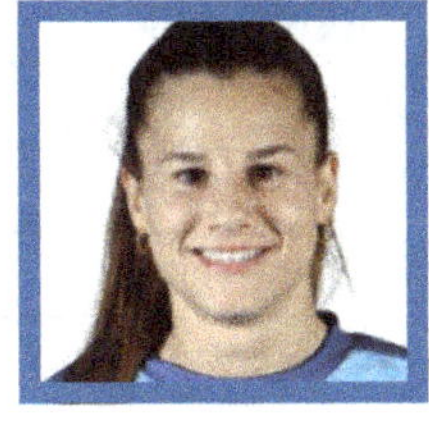

Elisa Del Estal: Contribuisce con 6 reti alla permanenza in A del club partenopeo

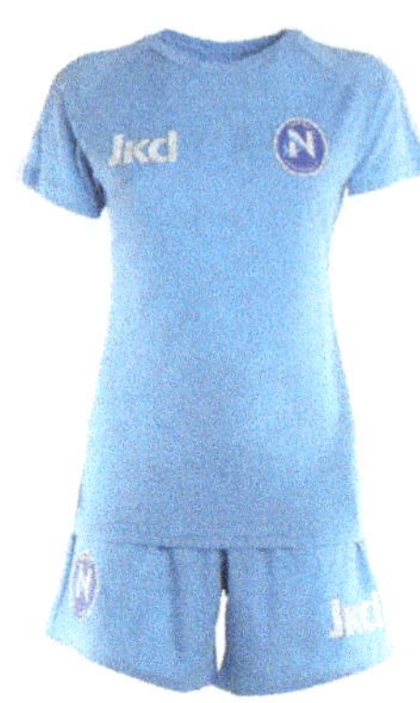

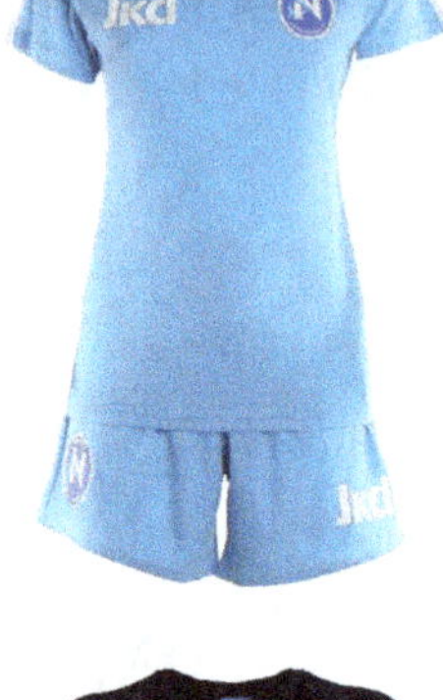

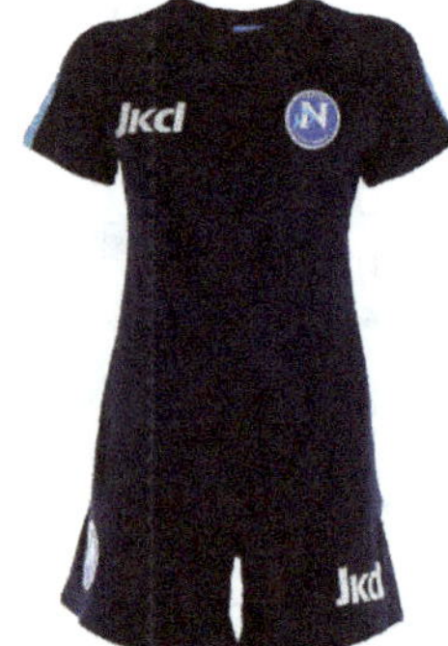

IL COMMENTO DELLA STAGIONE

Il neopromosso Napoli centra una sofferta salvezza. Le azzurre riescono a cancellare lo zero in classifica soltanto all'undicesima giornata, a vincere la prima partita a metà febbraio e ad avere la certezza di evitare la retrocessione diretta soltanto al penultimo turno della Poule Salvezza a seguito del pari contro il Milan e al contemporaneo ko del Pomigliano contro il Como. La squadra diretta da Biagio Seno si garantisce la permanenza in Serie A nello spareggio contro la Ternana (seconda in Serie B) vincendo la gara di andata in trasferta per 2-1 e pareggiando quella di ritorno in casa per 0-0. A fornire un contributo prezioso al raggiungimento dell'obiettivo è l'avanti Elisa Del Estal.

ANDAMENTO IN CAMPIONATO

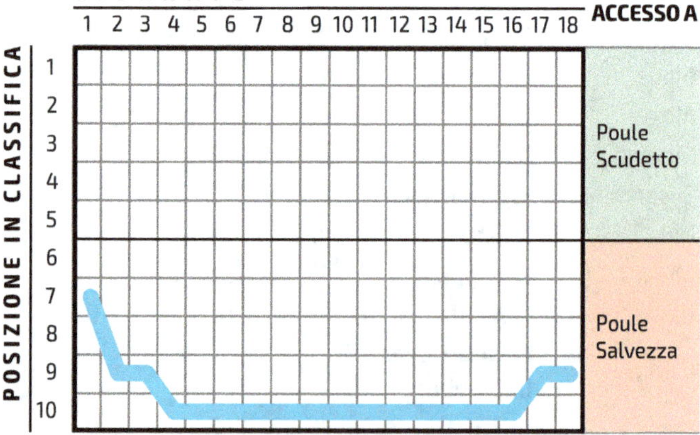

COMPORTAMENTO DELLA SQUADRA

Statistiche		Classifica	Rank
		10 09 08 07 06 05 04 03 02 01	
Giocatrici schierate	21		10
Giocatrici in rete	7		9
Giocatrici under 18	4		5
Giocatrici over 30	9		5
Cartellini gialli	33		10
Cartellini rossi	0		1
Cambi effettuati	66		9

LA STAGIONE 2023/2024

	Avversario	Casa / Fuori	Risultato		Arbitro
			Vinta Nulla Persa		
PRIMA FASE					
1	**Como Women**	F	2-1	Persa	Silvia Gasperotti
2	**Milan Femminile**	C	0-1	Persa	Mauro Gangi
3	**Fiorentina Femminile**	F	2-0	Persa	Luca Cherchi
4	**Sampdoria Femminile**	C	0-2	Persa	Adolfo Baratta
5	**Inter Women**	F	2-0	Persa	Antonino Costanza
6	**Sassuolo Femminile**	C	0-1	Persa	Cristiano Ursini
7	**Roma Femminile**	F	6-0	Persa	Luca De Angeli
8	**Pomigliano Femminile**	F	2-1	Persa	Valerio Crezzini
9	**Juventus Women**	C	1-3	Persa	Samuele Andreano
10	**Como Women**	C	0-0	Nulla	Simone Galipo
11	**Milan Femminile**	F	1-1	Nulla	Giuseppe Maria Manzo
12	**Fiorentina Femminile**	C	2-4	Persa	Erminio Cerbasi
13	**Sampdoria Femminile**	F	0-0	Nulla	Emanuele Ceriello
14	**Inter Women**	C	2-3	Persa	Gabriele Sacchi
15	**Sassuolo Femminile**	F	2-0	Persa	Antonio Di Reda
16	**Roma Femminile**	C	0-1	Persa	Francesco Zago
17	**Pomigliano Femminile**	C	2-0	Vinta	Giuseppe Mucera
18	**Juventus Women**	F	4-1	Persa	Giorgio Bozzetto
POULE SALVEZZA					
1	**Como Women**	F	1-1	Nulla	Mattia Nigro
3	**Sampdoria Femminile**	C	2-0	Vinta	Giuseppe Vingo
4	**Milan Femminile**	F	3-2	Persa	Gabriele Totaro
5	**Pomigliano Femminile**	C	1-1	Nulla	Marco Di Loreto
6	**Como Women**	C	1-1	Nulla	Emanuele Ceriello
8	**Sampdoria Femminile**	F	2-0	Persa	Andrea Zoppi
9	**Milan Femminile**	C	1-1	Nulla	Giorgio Di Cicco
10	**Pomigliano Femminile**	F	3-1	Persa	Silvia Gasperotti

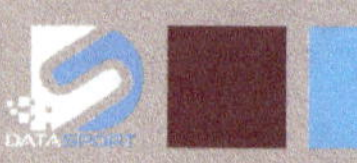

POMIGLIANO FEMMINILE

Pomigliano Calcio Femminile S.r.l.

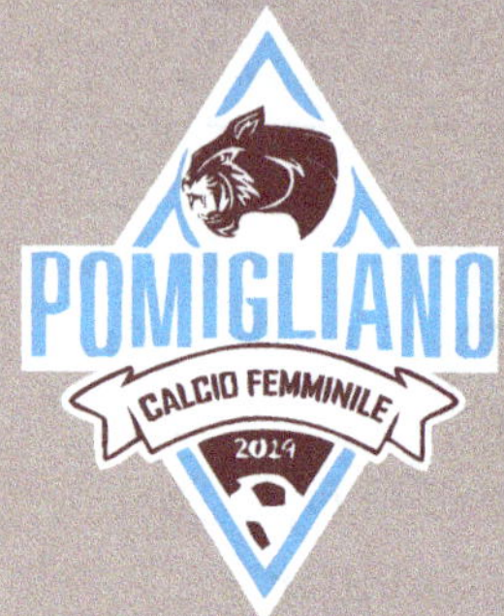

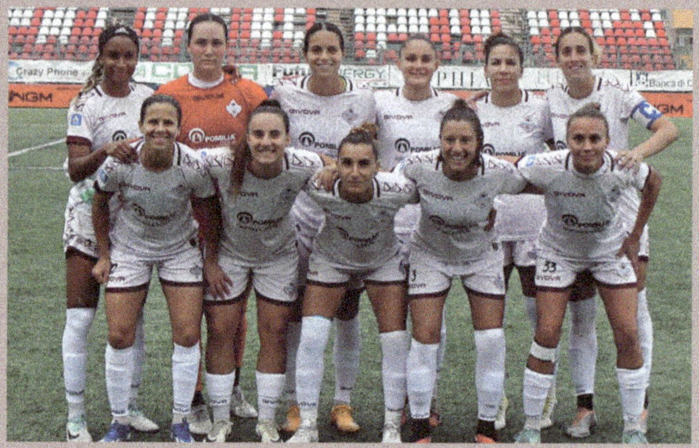

2019

Granata

Via Ravenna -
80038 Pomigliano
d'Arco (NA)

Amerigo Liguori
- Viale Ungheria,
54 - 80059 Torre
del Greco (NA)

ORGANIGRAMMA

Presidente Raffaele Pipola.
Vice Presidente Felice Pipola.
General manager Giuseppe Casertano.
Direttore sportivo Clemente Santonastaso.

STAFF TECNICO

Allenatore Antonio Contreras Olivera (1-6), Alessandro Caruso (7-16), Roberto Carannante.
Allenatore in seconda Gerardo Alfano.
Collaboratori tecnici Alessandro Riccio.
Preparatori atletici Ciro Zampella.
Preparatore dei portieri Giovanni Russo

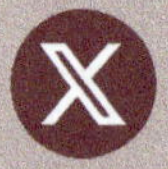

PROFILO X

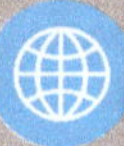

SITO INTERNET
pomiglianocalcio
femminile.it

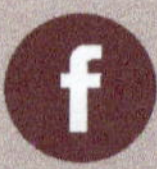

PAGINA FACEBOOK
PomiglianoWomen/

PROFILO INSTAGRAM
pomiglianowomen/

LA ROSA DELLA SQUADRA

Nome	Cognome	Nato il	PR	RE	AM	ES	SF	SA	Ruolo
Gaia	**Apicella**	28/10/1993	23	1	5	1	2	0	DIF
Nicole	**Arcangeli**	23/10/2003	13	3	1	0	1	4	ATT
Milica	**Babic**	05/06/2005	4	0	0	0	4	0	ATT
Elena	**Battistini**	10/08/2003	18	0	2	0	5	4	DIF
Laura	**Bourgoin**	17/09/1992	10	0	2	0	4	5	ATT
Anna Rosa James	**Buhigas**	16/12/1994	14	0	2	0	1	0	POR
Sara	**Caiazzo**	22/04/2003	23	0	0	0	0	1	DIF
Heden	**Corrado**	05/03/2002	6	0	0	0	4	0	DIF
Virginia	**Di Giammarino**	21/02/1999	26	0	4	0	0	18	CEN
Greis	**Domi**	30/10/1998	17	0	0	0	16	1	CEN
Zhanna	**Ferrario**	22/09/1993	24	3	1	0	1	6	CEN
Martina	**Fusini**	30/01/1996	23	0	3	0	2	9	DIF
Emilie	**Gavillet**	08/02/2000	13	0	0	0	0	0	POR
Aryana	**Harvey Lynn**	02/04/1997	21	1	3	0	2	7	DIF
Miriam	**Illiano**	05/09/2006	1	0	0	0	1	0	CEN
Dalila Belen	**Ippolito**	24/03/2002	20	3	3	0	1	8	ATT
Chiara	**Manca**	28/04/2001	11	1	0	0	11	0	ATT
Ana Lucia	**Martinez Maldonado**	08/01/1990	11	3	1	0	1	1	ATT
Violah	**Nambi**	24/07/1995	26	1	2	0	10	11	ATT
Debora	**Novellino**	11/09/1997	21	1	4	0	8	7	DIF
Iris	**Rabot**	16/10/2000	26	2	2	0	0	5	CEN
Sara	**Schettino**	12/01/2004	2	0	0	0	2	0	DIF
Marianela	**Szymanowski**	31/07/1990	18	2	1	0	9	2	CEN
Irina	**Talle**	16/04/2004	1	0	0	0	1	0	CEN
Lucie Murielle Dominique	**Tengue**	09/08/2001	1	0	0	0	1	0	ATT
Anna	**Vingiani**	09/02/2006	2	0	0	0	2	0	DIF

LEGENDA PR presenze - **RE** reti - **A** ammonizioni - **E** espulsioni - **SF** sostituzioni fatte - **SA** sostituzioni avute

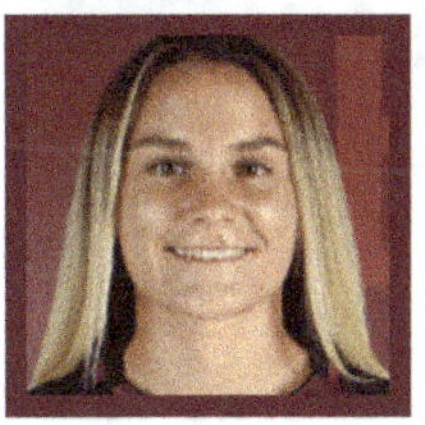

Iris Rabot: Come Di Giammarino e Nambi prende parte ai 26 match della sua squadra

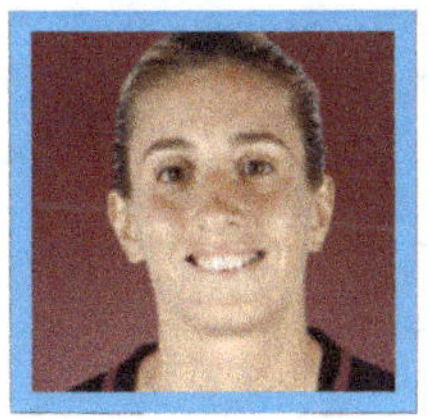

Gaia Apicella: Record di presenze (21) e reti (una) nella quinta stagione in granata

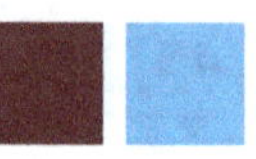

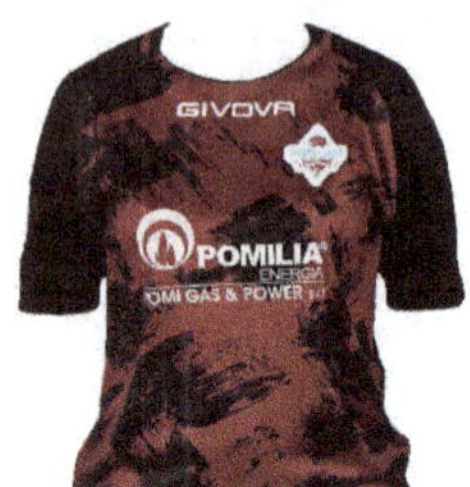

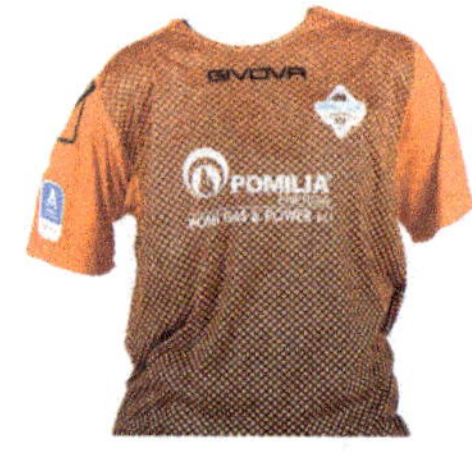

IL COMMENTO DELLA STAGIONE

Il Pomigliano abbandona dopo tre anni la Serie A. La formazione campana inizia il campionato raccogliendo un solo punto nelle prime sei gare. L'arrivo in panchina di Alessandro Caruso al posto di Antonio Contreras illude in merito a una possibile risalita delle granata. Il Pomigliano, dopo il successo sul Napoli e il pari contro il Como, consegue soltanto un punto in tutto il girone di ritorno chiudendo all'ultimo posto la regular season. Roberto Carannante, subentrato nel frattempo alla guida della squadra, non riesce a fare meglio dei suoi predecessori. La 2ª vittoria stagionale, ottenuta sempre sul Napoli, arriva nel match conclusivo della Poule Salvezza a retrocessione diretta già certa.

ANDAMENTO IN CAMPIONATO

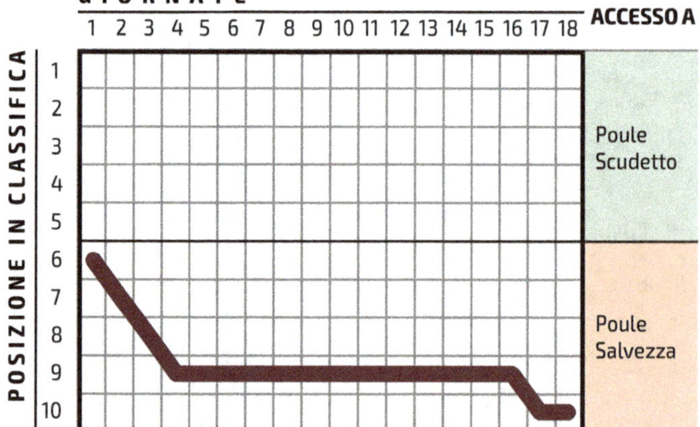

COMPORTAMENTO DELLA SQUADRA

Statistiche		Classifica	Rank
		10 09 08 07 06 05 04 03 02 01	
Giocatrici schierate	24	██ ██	9
Giocatrici in rete	8	██ ██ ██ ██ ██	6
Giocatrici under 18	5	██ ██ ██ ██ ██ ██ ██	4
Giocatrici over 30	8	██ ██ ██ ██ ██	6
Cartellini gialli	29	██ ██ ██	8
Cartellini rossi	1	██ ██ ██ ██ ██	6
Cambi effettuati	67	██ ██ ██	8

LA STAGIONE 2023/2024

	Avversario	Casa / Fuori	Risultato		Arbitro
PRIMA FASE					
1	**Juventus Women**	C	2-3	Persa	Gabriele Totaro
2	**Sassuolo Femminile**	F	1-1	Nulla	Gianluca Renzi
3	**Roma Femminile**	C	0-5	Persa	Antonio Di Reda
4	**Fiorentina Femminile**	C	1-4	Persa	Dario Di Francesco
5	**Milan Femminile**	F	4-1	Persa	Gabriele Sacchi
6	**Sampdoria Femminile**	C	0-1	Persa	Luigi Catanoso
7	**Inter Women**	F	2-1	Persa	Stefano Nicolini
8	**Napoli Femminile**	C	2-1	Vinta	Valerio Crezzini
9	**Como Women**	F	0-0	Nulla	Ermes F. Cavaliere
10	**Juventus Women**	F	4-0	Persa	Mattia Caldera
11	**Sassuolo Femminile**	C	0-2	Persa	Valerio Vogliacco
12	**Roma Femminile**	F	3-0	Persa	Jules R. A. Tona Mbei
13	**Fiorentina Femminile**	F	3-1	Persa	Simone Gavini
14	**Milan Femminile**	C	0-0	Nulla	Domenico Leone
15	**Sampdoria Femminile**	F	1-0	Persa	Enrico Gigliotti
16	**Inter Women**	C	2-6	Persa	Mario Perri
17	**Napoli Femminile**	F	2-0	Persa	Giuseppe Mucera
18	**Como Women**	C	3-4	Persa	Valerio Pezzopane
POULE SALVEZZA					
1	**Sampdoria Femminile**	C	0-5	Persa	Felipe S. Viapiana
2	**Milan Femminile**	F	4-0	Persa	Jules R. A. Tona Mbei
4	**Como Women**	C	1-2	Persa	Gabriele Restaldo
5	**Napoli Femminile**	F	1-1	Nulla	Marco Di Loreto
6	**Sampdoria Femminile**	F	2-2	Nulla	Giorgio Di Cicco
7	**Milan Femminile**	C	2-2	Nulla	Adolfo Baratta
9	**Como Women**	F	2-0	Persa	Gioele Iacobellis
10	**Napoli Femminile**	C	3-1	Vinta	Silvia Gasperotti

ROMA FEMMINILE

AS Roma S.r.l.

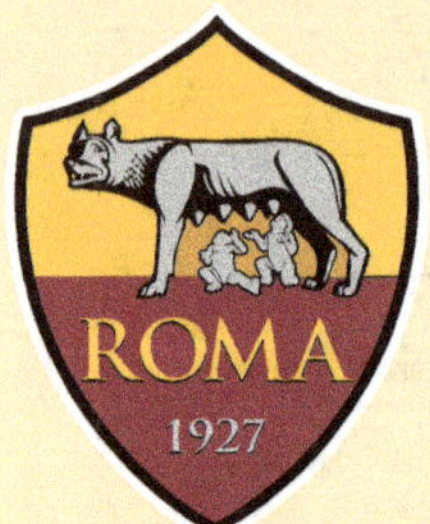

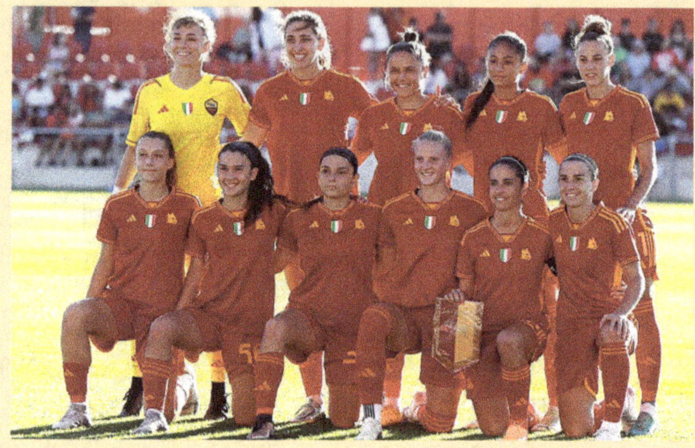

ANNO DI FONDAZIONE
2018

COLORI SOCIALI
Giallo Rosso

INDIRIZZO SEDE
Piazzale Dino Viola, 1 - 00128 Roma

STADIO
Tre Fontane - Via delle Tre Fontane, 6 - 00144 Roma

ORGANIGRAMMA

Presidente Dan Friedkin.
Direttore settore femminile Elisabetta Bavagnoli.
Team manager Ilaria Inchingolo.

STAFF TECNICO

Allenatore Alessandro Spugna.
Allenatore in seconda Leonardo Montesano.
Collaboratori tecnici Riccardo Ciocchetti.
Preparatori atletici Stefano D'Ottavio, Simone Mangieri, Davide Massimi, Fiore Coli.
Preparatore dei portieri Mauro Patrizi

PROFILO X
ASRomaFemminile/

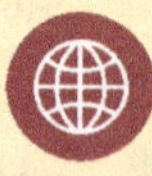

SITO INTERNET
asroma.com

PAGINA FACEBOOK
officialasroma

PROFILO INSTAGRAM
asromawomen/

LA ROSA DELLA SQUADRA

Nome	Cognome	Nato il	PR	RE	AM	ES	SF	SA	Ruolo
Eseosa	**Aigbogun**	23/05/1993	10	0	2	0	1	1	DIF
Elisa	**Bartoli**	07/05/1991	16	0	1	1	2	2	DIF
Camelia	**Ceasar**	13/12/1997	19	0	1	0	0	0	POR
Claudia	**Ciccotti**	09/02/1994	6	0	0	0	5	1	CEN
Lucia	**Di Guglielmo**	26/06/1997	19	4	3	0	4	6	DIF
Laura	**Feiersinger**	05/04/1993	23	4	0	0	17	3	CEN
Aurora	**Galli**	13/12/1996	1	0	0	0	1	0	CEN
Valentina	**Giacinti**	02/01/1994	26	12	3	0	6	16	ATT
Manuela	**Giugliano**	18/08/1997	25	10	2	0	1	16	CEN
Benedetta	**Glionna**	26/07/1999	18	3	0	0	9	8	ATT
Giada	**Greggi**	18/02/2000	24	4	1	0	4	15	CEN
Emilie	**Haavi**	16/06/1992	25	3	0	0	1	14	ATT
Tinja-Riikka	**Korpela**	05/05/1986	7	0	0	0	1	0	POR
Zara	**Kramzar**	10/01/2006	7	1	0	0	5	1	CEN
Saki	**Kumagai**	17/10/1990	25	5	2	0	2	7	CEN
Barbara	**Latorre**	14/03/1993	8	0	0	0	5	3	ATT
Elena	**Linari**	15/04/1994	22	7	2	0	0	1	DIF
Moeka	**Minami**	07/12/1998	24	1	3	0	1	0	DIF
Stephanie	**Ohrstrom**	12/01/1987	1	0	0	0	0	1	POR
Giada	**Pellegrino Cimo**	07/10/2006	3	0	0	0	3	0	ATT
Alayah	**Pilgrim**	29/04/2003	10	1	0	0	7	3	ATT
Anja	**Sonstevold**	21/06/1992	13	0	0	0	2	1	DIF
Annamaria	**Serturini**	13/05/1998	8	0	1	0	8	0	ATT
Martina	**Tomaselli**	01/08/2001	13	2	0	0	11	2	CEN
Sanne	**Troelsgaard**	15/08/1988	12	2	1	0	10	1	CEN
Oihane	**Valdezate**	10/04/2000	11	1	1	0	3	2	DIF
Evelyne	**Viens**	06/02/1997	24	13	2	0	5	10	ATT

LEGENDA PR presenze - **RE** reti - **A** ammonizioni - **E** espulsioni - **SF** sostituzioni fatte - **SA** sostituzioni avute

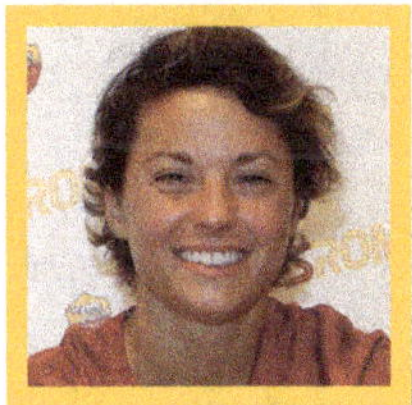

Valentina Giacinti: Seconda nella classifica marcatori (12 gol) e in quella degli assist (7)

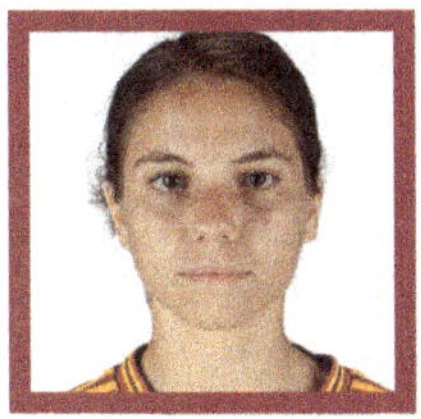

Manuela Giugliano: La capitana giallorossa chiude il torneo con 10 reti e 7 assist

41

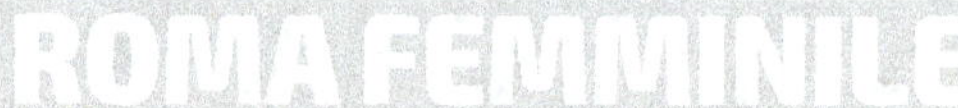

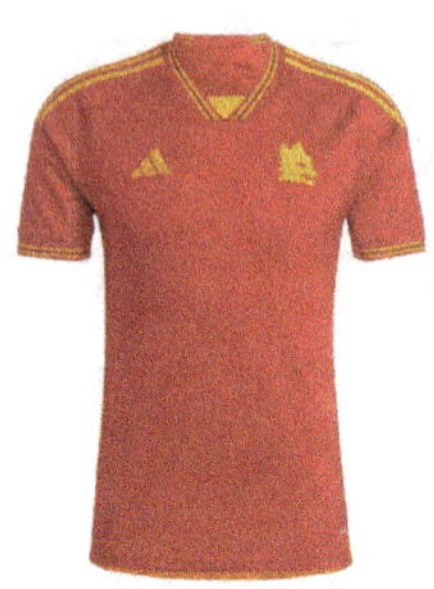

IL COMMENTO DELLA STAGIONE

La Roma si conferma Campione d'Italia con un bilancio finale di 26 vittorie, un pari e 2 sconfitte. Le giallorosse conquistano il loro secondo titolo con quattro giornate d'anticipo sul termine della Poule Scudetto. La formazione diretta da Alessandro Spugna, dopo aver chiuso al comando la regular season con otto punti di vantaggio sulla Juventus, incrementa il divario nella seconda fase portandolo a undici lunghezze. Tra le artefici del trionfo, maturato con l'attacco più prolifico e variegato (sedici marcatrici diverse) e la difesa meno battuta, meritano una citazione particolare la centrocampista Manuela Giugliano e le avanti Evelyne Viens (capocannoniere del torneo) e Valentina Giacinti.

ANDAMENTO IN CAMPIONATO

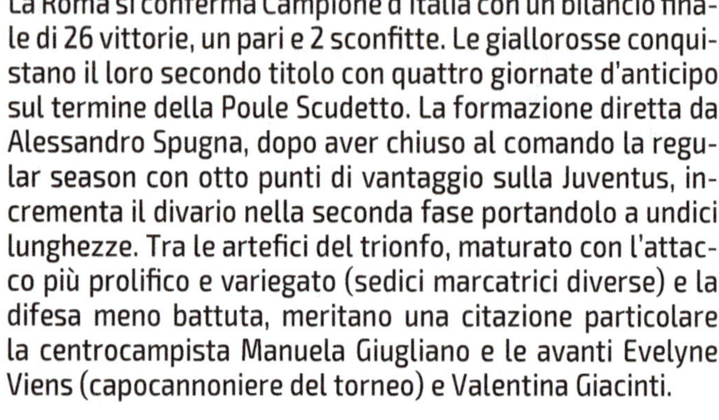

COMPORTAMENTO DELLA SQUADRA

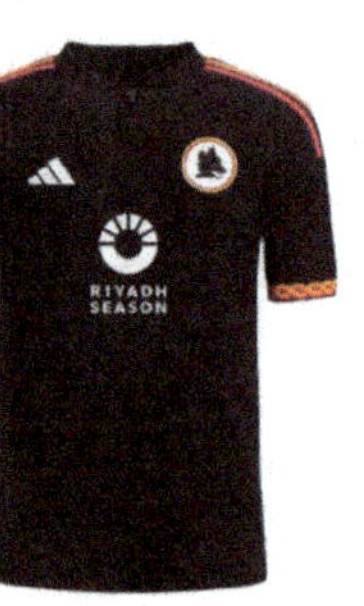

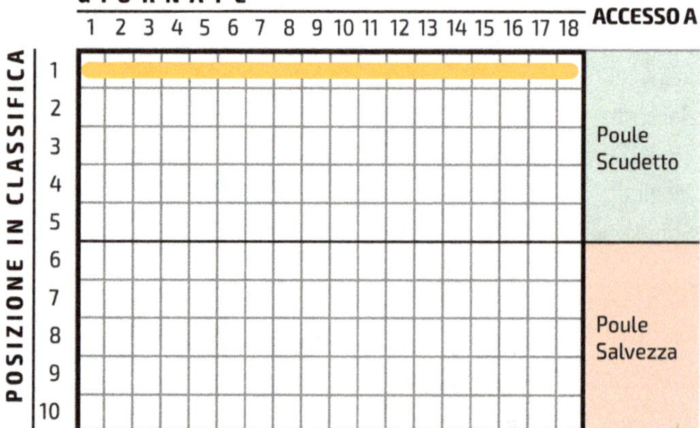

Statistiche		Classifica	Rank
		10 09 08 07 06 05 04 03 02 01	
Giocatrici schierate	25		6
Giocatrici in rete	13		1
Giocatrici under 18	4		5
Giocatrici over 30	19		1
Cartellini gialli	16		1
Cartellini rossi	1		6
Cambi effettuati	79		4

LA STAGIONE 2023/2024

	Avversario	Casa / Fuori	Risultato		Arbitro
			Vinta · Nulla · Persa		
PRIMA FASE					
1	**Milan Femminile**	F	2-4	Vinta	Domenico Castellone
2	**Como Women**	C	4-1	Vinta	Gabriele Totaro
3	**Pomigliano Femminile**	F	0-5	Vinta	Antonio Di Reda
4	**Inter Women**	C	2-0	Vinta	Marco Emmanuele
5	**Sampdoria Femminile**	F	0-5	Vinta	Lorenzo Maccarini
6	**Juventus Women**	F	1-3	Vinta	Domenico Mirabella
7	**Napoli Femminile**	C	6-0	Vinta	Luca De Angeli
8	**Sassuolo Femminile**	F	0-2	Vinta	Gianluca Renzi
9	**Fiorentina Femminie**	C	2-1	Vinta	Silvia Gasperotti
10	**Milan Femminile**	C	2-1	Vinta	Filippo Giaccaglia
11	**Como Women**	F	2-3	Vinta	Mattia Nigro
12	**Pomigliano Femminile**	C	3-0	Vinta	Jules R. A. Tona Mbei
13	**Inter Women**	F	2-0	Persa	Samuele Andreano
14	**Sampdoria Femminile**	C	2-0	Vinta	Cristiano Ursini
15	**Juventus Women**	C	3-1	Vinta	Marco Emmanuele
16	**Napoli Femminile**	F	0-1	Vinta	Francesco Zago
17	**Sassuolo Femminile**	C	3-0	Vinta	Daniele Virgilio
18	**Fiorentina Femminie**	F	0-1	Vinta	Giorgio Vergaro
POULE SCUDETTO					
2	**Sassuolo Femminile**	C	3-0	Vinta	Maria Marotta
3	**Inter Women**	F	1-2	Vinta	Andrea Zanotti
4	**Juventus Women**	C	2-1	Vinta	Lorenzo Maccarini
5	**Fiorentina Femminile**	F	0-0	Nulla	Carlo Rinaldi
7	**Sassuolo Femminile**	F	5-6	Vinta	Fabrizio Ramondino
8	**Inter Women**	C	4-3	Vinta	Giuseppe Maria Manzo
9	**Juventus Women**	F	3-1	Persa	Cristiano Ursini
10	**Fiorentina Femminile**	C	5-0	Vinta	Valerio Vogliacco

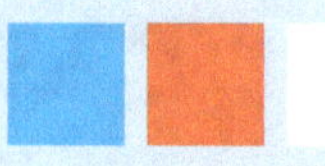

SAMPDORIA FEMMINILE
UC Sampdoria Women S.p.A.

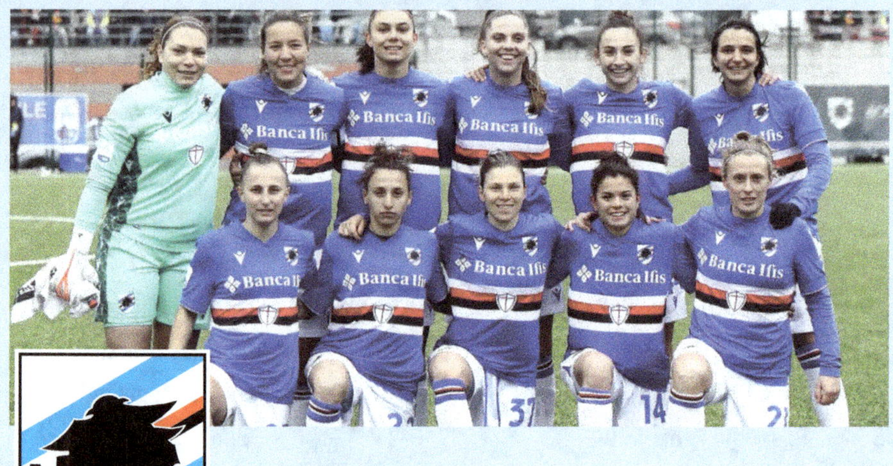

Presidente Marco Lanna.
Responsabile Sampdoria Women Marco Palmieri.
Segretaria Marcella Ghilardi.

ANNO DI FONDAZIONE
2020

COLORI SOCIALI
Blu Bianco
Rosso Nero

INDIRIZZO SEDE
Piazza Borgo Pila,
39 (Torre B - 5°
piano) - 16129
Genova

STAFF TECNICO
Allenatore Salvatore Mango (1-21), Gian Loris Rossi.
Allenatrice Stefano Castiglione.
Allenatore in seconda Marco Ferri.
Preparatori atletici Bartolomeo Segale.
Preparatore dei portieri Fabrizio Casazza

STADIO
La Sciorba - Via Gelasio Adamoli, 57 - Genova

PROFILO X
sampdoria/

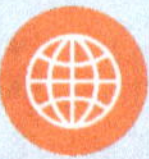

SITO INTERNET
sampdoria.it

PAGINA FACEBOOK
sampdoria/

PROFILO INSTAGRAM
sampdoria/

LA ROSA DELLA SQUADRA

Nome	Cognome	Nato il	PR	RE	AM	ES	SF	SA	Ruolo
Sara	**Baldi**	13/04/2000	13	2	2	0	4	7	ATT
Veronica	**Battelani**	23/07/2002	17	0	3	0	10	7	CEN
Alice	**Benoit**	27/03/1996	25	0	4	0	1	9	CEN
Asia	**Bragonzi**	05/03/2001	9	1	1	0	7	1	ATT
Martina	**Brustia**	04/07/1998	7	0	2	0	2	3	CEN
Rachel	**Cuschieri**	26/04/1992	24	0	1	0	6	16	CEN
Aurora	**De Rita**	22/10/1999	24	2	4	0	0	6	DIF
Talia	**Della Peruta T.**	19/04/2002	10	1	0	0	5	4	CEN
Victoria Marie	**Della Peruta V.**	21/03/2004	11	8	1	0	6	1	ATT
Bianca	**Fallico**	04/08/1999	10	0	0	0	8	1	CEN
Michela	**Giordano**	29/08/2002	25	2	1	0	2	14	DIF
Nora	**Heroum**	20/07/1994	22	0	0	0	11	4	DIF
Sarah	**Huchet**	04/05/1994	8	0	2	0	4	2	CEN
Kettu	**Karresmaa**	22/08/2004	4	0	1	0	0	0	POR
Giada	**Lopez Toaquiza**	14/03/2005	1	0	0	0	1	0	ATT
Chiara	**Marenco**	12/05/2004	3	0	0	0	3	0	DIF
Chiara	**Micheli**	26/06/2002	2	0	0	0	2	0	DIF
Virag	**Nagy**	04/07/2001	5	0	1	0	5	0	DIF
Elisabetta	**Oliviero**	18/07/1997	26	0	2	0	0	2	DIF
Vanessa	**Panzeri**	22/06/2000	3	0	0	0	0	0	DIF
Elena	**Pisani**	12/11/1997	20	0	1	0	1	2	DIF
Cecilia	**Re**	28/03/1994	24	1	8	0	1	0	CEN
Syria	**Rosignoli**	28/02/2006	1	0	0	0	1	0	ATT
Eva	**Schatzer**	16/01/2005	23	2	0	0	1	4	CEN
Alice Karin	**Sondergaard**	22/05/2003	6	0	1	0	4	2	ATT
Amanda	**Tampieri**	11/02/1997	22	0	1	0	0	0	POR
Stefania	**Tarenzi**	29/02/1988	13	1	0	0	7	5	ATT
Cristina Sena das Neves	**Tatiely**	11/08/1996	22	4	5	0	2	4	ATT

LEGENDA PR presenze - **RE** reti - **A** ammonizioni - **E** espulsioni - **SF** sostituzioni fatte - **SA** sostituzioni avute

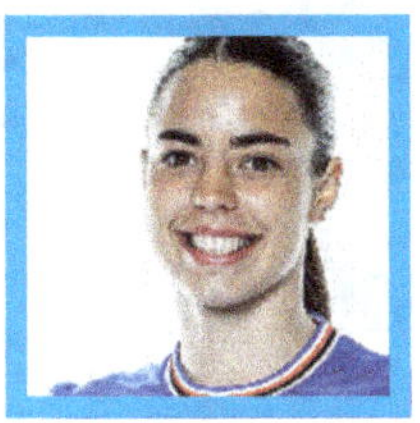

Victoria Della Peruta: La 20enne blucerchiata brilla andando a segno ogni 70 minuti

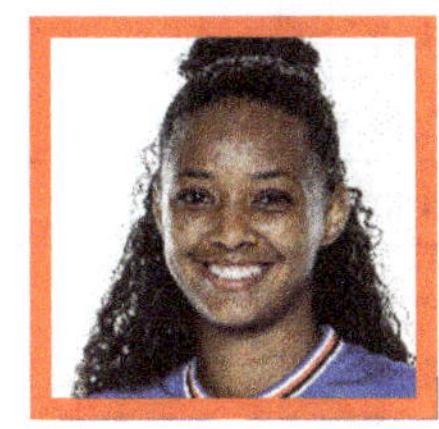

Tatiely Sena: La centrocampista brasiliana contribuisce alla salvezza: 4 gol e 2 assist

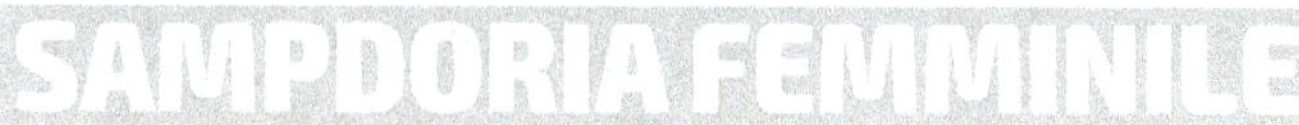

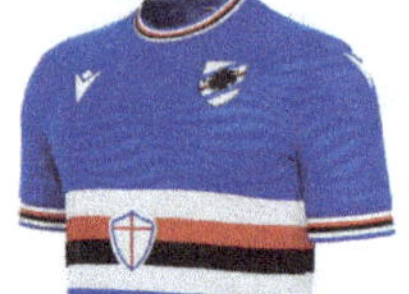

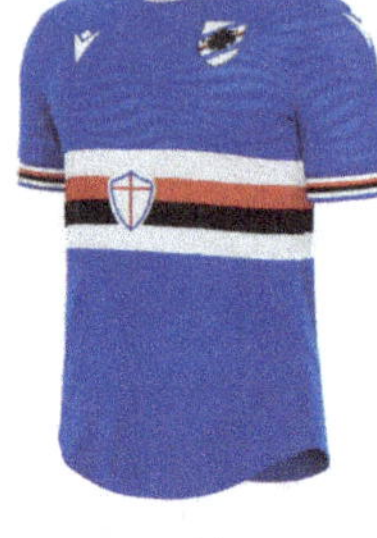

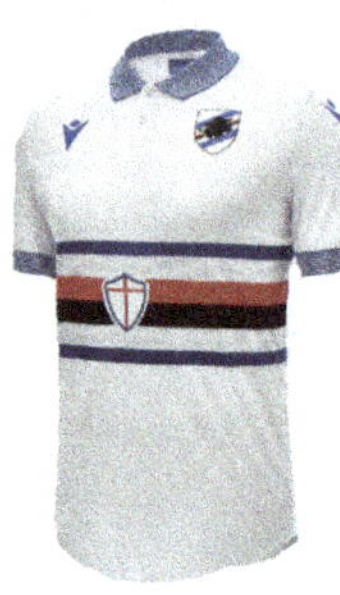

IL COMMENTO DELLA STAGIONE

La Sampdoria conferma l'ottavo posto della passata stagione centrando però l'obiettivo salvezza con meno patemi. Le blucerchiate, dopo aver racimolato 7 punti nel girone d'andata, ne conquistano 11 in quello di ritorno. Un bottino che consente alla compagine ligure di iniziare la Poule Salvezza con un rassicurante margine di dodici lunghezze sulle ultime della classe. Le affermazioni colte in avvio di seconda fase contro Pomigliano e Como permettono alla Sampdoria di conseguire con largo anticipo la permanenza nella serie maggiore. Sorprendentemente il tecnico Salvatore Mango viene avvicendato il 4 aprile con Gian Loris Rossi. Menzione particolare per la giovane Victoria Marie Della Peruta.

ANDAMENTO IN CAMPIONATO

COMPORTAMENTO DELLA SQUADRA

Statistiche		Classifica											Rank
		10	09	08	07	06	05	04	03	02	01		
Giocatrici schierate	26												3
Giocatrici in rete	7												9
Giocatrici under 18	6												3
Giocatrici over 30	8												6
Cartellini gialli	26												6
Cartellini rossi	0												1
Cambi effettuati	61												10

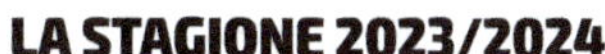

LA STAGIONE 2023/2024

	Avversario	Casa / Fuori	Risultato		Arbitro
			Vinta Nulla Persa		
PRIMA FASE					
1	**Inter Women**	C	0-2		Edoardo Gianquinto
2	**Juventus Women**	F	4-1		Luca De Angeli
3	**Como Women**	C	1-2		Edoardo M. Mazzoni
4	**Napoli Femminile**	F	0-2		Adolfo Baratta
5	**Roma Femminile**	C	0-5		Lorenzo Maccarini
6	**Pomigliano Femminile**	F	0-1		Luigi Catanoso
7	**Fiorentina Femminile**	C	0-1		Maria Marotta
8	**Milan Femminile**	F	1-1		Giuseppe C. Allegretta
9	**Sassuolo Femminile**	C	0-4		Filippo Colaninno
10	**Inter Women**	F	1-1		Aleksandar Djurdjevic
11	**Juventus Women**	C	1-0		Giorgio Bozzetto
12	**Como Women**	F	0-1		Enrico Cappai
13	**Napoli Femminile**	C	0-0		Emanuele Ceriello
14	**Roma Femminile**	F	2-0		Cristiano Ursini
15	**Pomigliano Femminile**	C	1-0		Enrico Gigliotti
16	**Fiorentina Femminile**	F	2-1		Filippo Colaninno
17	**Milan Femminile**	C	1-3		Simone Gauzolino
18	**Sassuolo Femminile**	F	2-0		Fabio Rosario Luongo
POULE SALVEZZA					
1	**Pomigliano Femminile**	F	0-5		Felipe S. Viapiana
2	**Como Women**	C	1-0		Gabriele Restaldo
3	**Napoli Femminile**	F	2-0		Giuseppe Vingo
5	**Milan Femminile**	C	1-3		Edoardo M. Mazzoni
6	**Pomigliano Femminile**	C	2-2		Giorgio Di Cicco
7	**Como Women**	F	3-1		Alberto Poli
8	**Napoli Femminile**	C	2-0		Andrea Zoppi
10	**Milan Femminile**	F	3-1		Davide Gandino

SASSUOLO FEMMINILE

US Sassuolo Calcio s.r.l.

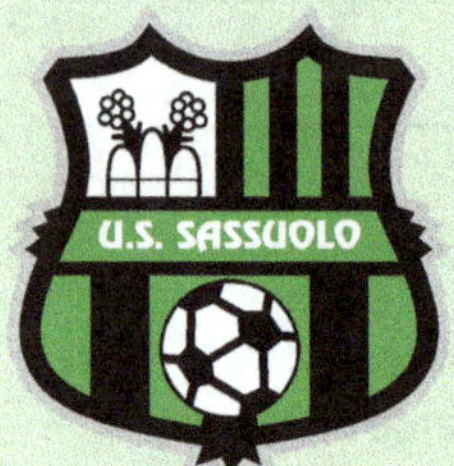

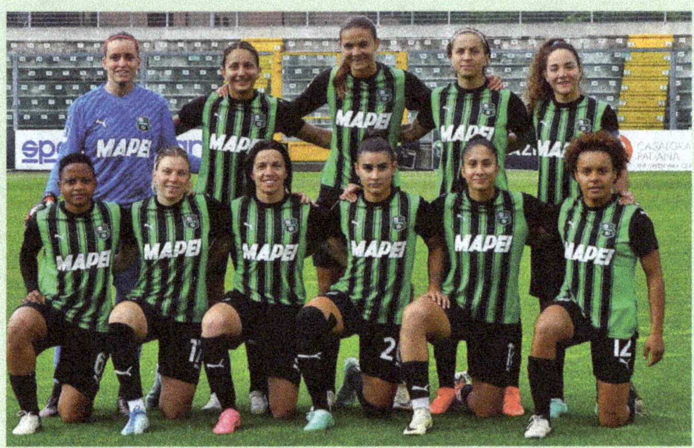

2016

Nero Verde

Via Giorgio Squinzi, 1 - 41049 Sassuolo (MO)

Enzo Ricci - Piazza Risorgimento, 47 - 41049 Sassuolo (MO)

ORGANIGRAMMA

Presidente Betty Vignotto.
Direttore sviluppo area calcio femminile Alessandro Terzi.
Team manager Annalisa Ielli.

STAFF TECNICO

Allenatore Gianpiero Piovani.
Allenatore in seconda Stefano Sacchetti.
Preparatori atletici Matteo Benassi, Ilaria Lancellotti.
Preparatore dei portieri Raffaele Nuzzo.
Match analyst Giulio Sciascia.

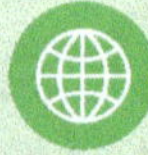

PROFILO X
SassuoloUS/

SITO INTERNET
sassuolocalcio.it/ femminile/

PAGINA FACEBOOK
officialsassuolo calcio/

PROFILO INSTAGRAM
sassuolocalcio/

Nome	Cognome	Nato il	PR	RE	AM	ES	SF	SA	Ruolo
Chiara	**Beccari**	27/09/2004	21	5	3	0	5	12	ATT
Benedetta	**Brignoli**	04/10/1999	13	0	1	0	5	5	CEN
Martina	**Brustia**	04/07/1998	1	0	0	0	1	0	CEN
Lana	**Clelland**	26/01/1993	21	9	0	0	5	13	ATT
Solene	**Durand**	20/11/1994	24	0	1	0	1	0	POR
Anastasia	**Ferrara**	24/10/2004	2	0	0	0	2	0	CEN
Maria Luisa	**Filangeri**	28/01/2000	25	0	5	0	0	2	DIF
Refiloe	**Jane**	04/08/1992	7	0	0	0	2	4	CEN
Isabella	**Kresche**	28/11/1998	2	0	0	0	0	1	POR
Loreta	**Kullashi**	20/05/1999	25	7	2	0	10	11	ATT
Lia	**Lonni**	17/01/2000	1	0	0	0	0	0	POR
Sara	**Mella**	14/04/1998	11	0	2	0	3	3	DIF
Naja Poje	**Mihelic**	17/08/2006	12	0	1	0	11	0	DIF
Kassandra Ndoutou E.	**Missipo**	03/02/1998	24	1	1	0	3	8	CEN
Valeria	**Monte-rubbiano**	27/07/1996	16	1	0	0	13	3	ATT
Virag	**Nagy**	04/07/2001	1	1	0	0	1	0	DIF
Benedetta	**Orsi**	25/02/2000	20	0	3	0	0	3	DIF
Angela	**Passeri**	21/07/2004	10	0	1	0	5	3	DIF
Davina	**Philtjens**	26/02/1989	24	0	1	0	1	3	DIF
Caroline Gram	**Pleidrup**	11/12/2000	26	1	3	0	0	1	DIF
Giada	**Pondini**	18/03/1997	24	0	0	0	2	17	CEN
Cecilia	**Prugna**	07/11/1997	21	2	1	0	7	6	CEN
Daniela	**Sabatino**	26/06/1985	24	7	0	0	6	10	ATT
Erika	**Santoro**	03/09/1999	14	0	1	1	8	3	DIF
Manuela	**Sciabica**	19/06/2006	11	2	2	0	10	1	ATT
Benedicte	**Simon**	02/06/1997	7	0	0	0	7	0	DIF
Giorgia	**Tudisco**	11/01/1995	3	0	0	0	3	0	CEN
Annahita	**Zamanian Le Loc'h Bakhtiari**	19/02/1998	11	2	0	0	4	6	CEN

LEGENDA PR presenze - **RE** reti - **A** ammonizioni - **E** espulsioni - **SF** sostituzioni fatte - **SA** sostituzioni avute

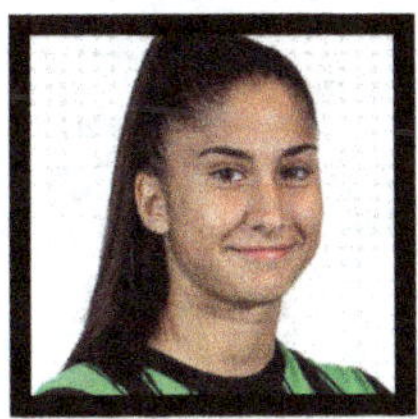

Chiara Beccari: Cinque reti e altrettanti assist per l'avanti del Sassuolo

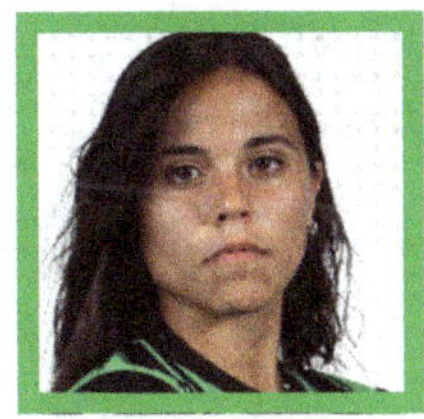

Giada Pontini: La veterana neroverde totalizza 24 presenze (22 da titolare)

IL COMMENTO DELLA STAGIONE

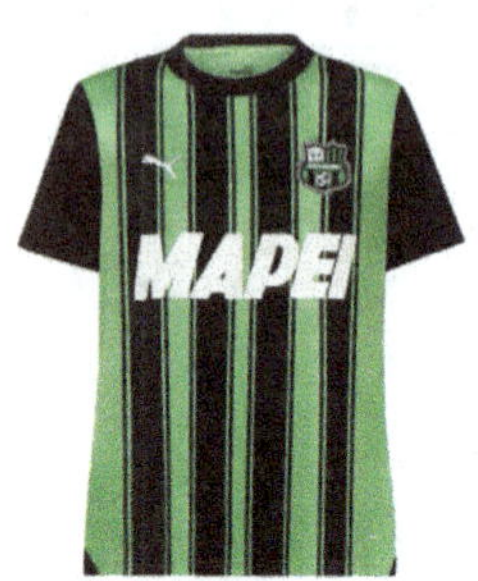

Campionato più che positivo quello disputato dal Sassuolo. La squadra guidata da Gianpiero Piovani, dopo un girone di andata avaro di soddisfazioni (solo 8 punti ottenuti), risale la classifica a suon di vittorie (6) chiudendo la regular season al quarto posto (due posizioni più su rispetto al 2022-23). Nella Poule Scudetto le neroverdi, continuando a giocare a viso aperto contro tutte le avversarie (da rammentare il ko interno per 5-6 contro la Roma) portano a casa dieci punti. Bottino che si rivela sufficiente per staccare l'Inter, ma non tale da impensierire la Fiorentina. Da sottolineare le prestazioni offerte in avanti da Chiara Beccari, Lana Clelland, Loreta Kullashi e Daniela Sabatino.

ANDAMENTO IN CAMPIONATO

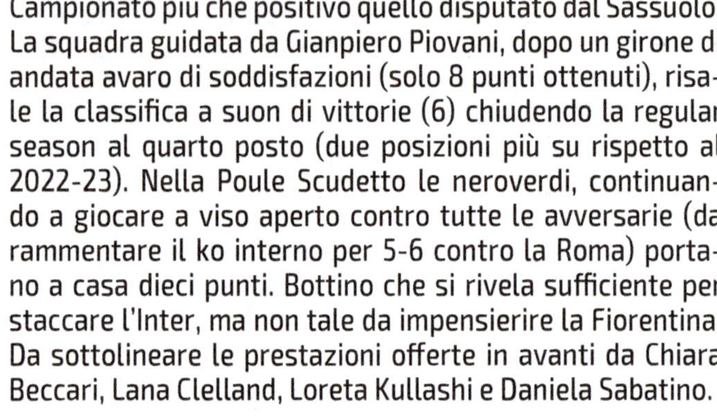

COMPORTAMENTO DELLA SQUADRA

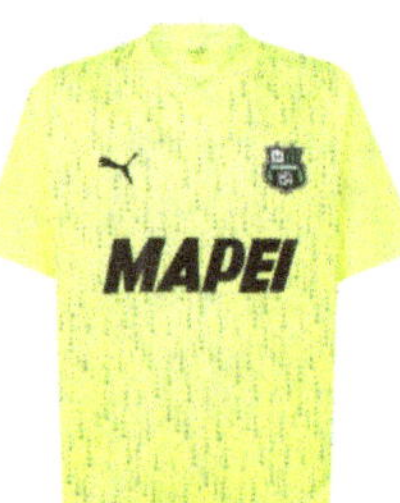

Statistiche		Classifica	Rank
		10 09 08 07 06 05 04 03 02 01	
Giocatrici schierate	28		1
Giocatrici in rete	8		6
Giocatrici under 18	3		7
Giocatrici over 30	5		10
Cartellini gialli	19		3
Cartellini rossi	1		6
Cambi effettuati	79		4

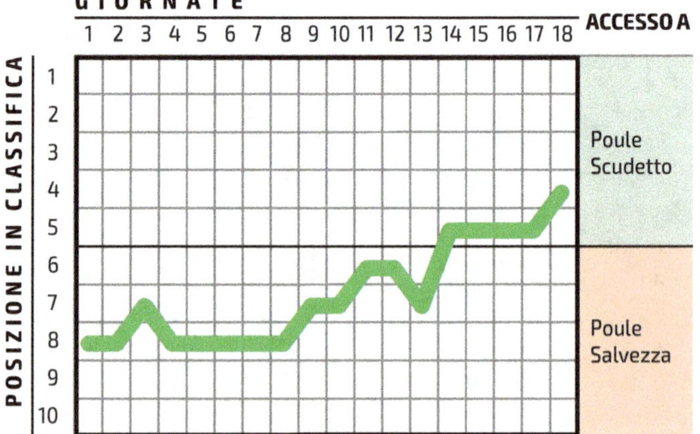

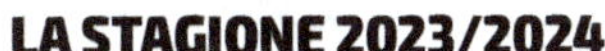

LA STAGIONE 2023/2024

	Avversario	Casa / Fuori	Risultato		Arbitro
PRIMA FASE					
1	**Fiorentina Femminile**	F	2-1	Persa	Juan Luca Sacchi
2	**Pomigliano Femminile**	C	1-1	Nulla	Gianluca Renzi
3	**Inter Women**	C	1-2	Persa	Simone Galipo
4	**Juventus Women**	F	4-0	Persa	Giuseppe Vingo
5	**Como Women**	C	1-2	Persa	Andrea Zoppi
6	**Napoli Femminile**	F	0-1	Vinta	Cristiano Ursini
7	**Milan Femminile**	F	1-1	Nulla	Carlo Rinaldi
8	**Roma Femminile**	C	0-2	Persa	Gianluca Renzi
9	**Sampdoria Femminile**	F	0-4	Vinta	Filippo Colaninno
10	**Fiorentina Femminile**	C	1-2	Persa	Gabriele Sacchi
11	**Pomigliano Femminile**	F	0-2	Vinta	Valerio Vogliacco
12	**Inter Women**	F	0-1	Vinta	Marco Peletti
13	**Juventus Women**	C	0-1	Persa	Andrea Ancora
14	**Como Women**	F	0-1	Vinta	Edoardo M. Mazzoni
15	**Napoli Femminile**	C	2-0	Vinta	Antonio Di Reda
16	**Milan Femminile**	C	1-0	Vinta	Eugenio Scarpa
17	**Roma Femminile**	F	3-0	Persa	Daniele Virgilio
18	**Sampdoria Femminile**	C	2-0	Vinta	Fabio Rosario Luongo
POULE SCUDETTO					
1	**Fiorentina Femminile**	C	1-0	Vinta	Alberto Poli
2	**Roma Femminile**	F	3-0	Persa	Maria Marotta
4	**Inter Women**	C	2-1	Vinta	Alessandro Silvestri
5	**Juventus Women**	F	2-1	Persa	Gianluca Renzi
6	**Fiorentina Femminile**	F	4-4	Nulla	Antonio Di Reda
7	**Roma Femminile**	C	5-6	Persa	Fabrizio Ramondino
9	**Inter Women**	F	2-4	Vinta	Francesco D'Eusanio
10	**Juventus Women**	C	2-3	Persa	Simone Gavini

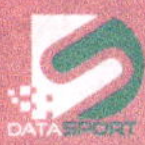

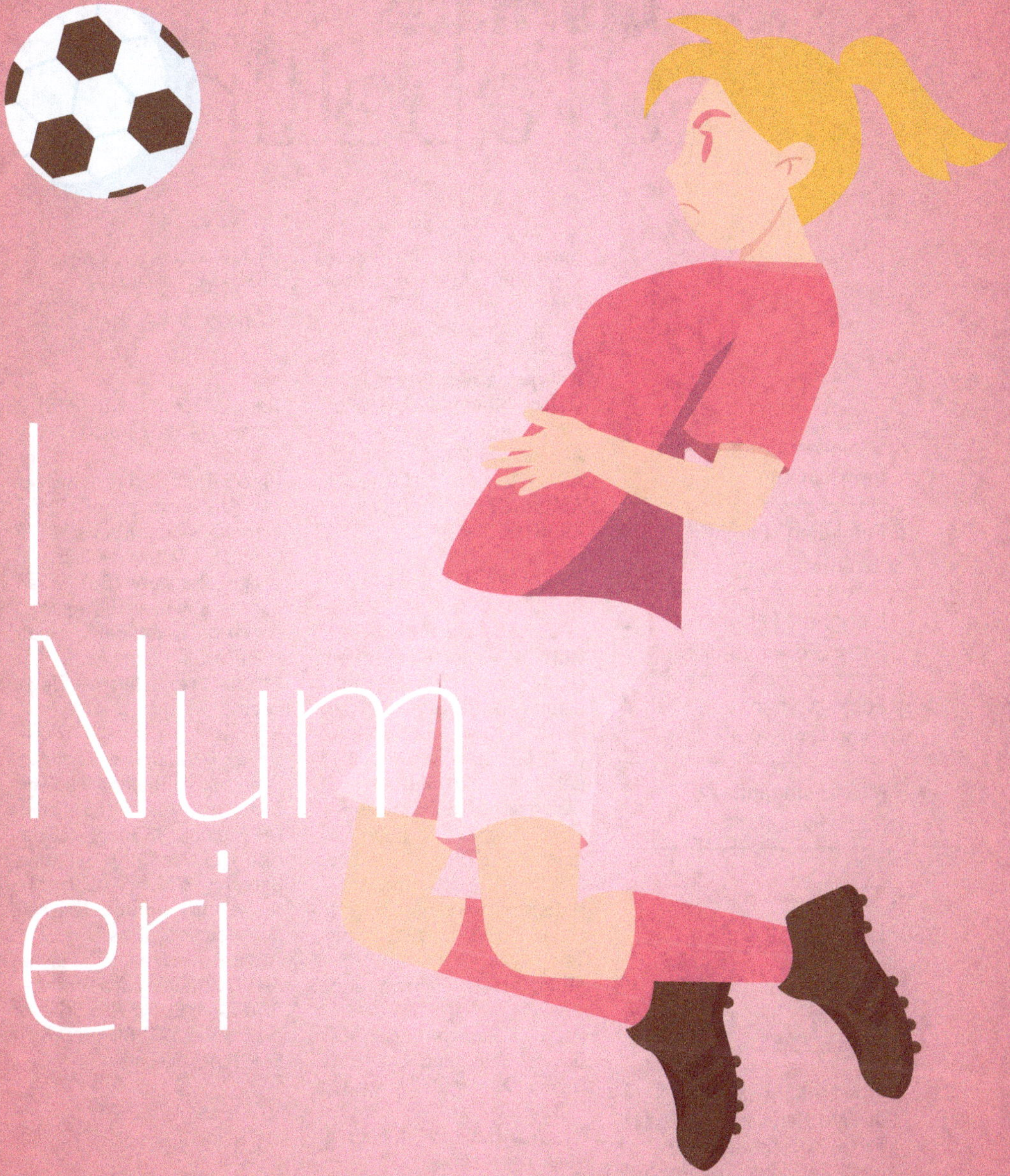

I Numeri

Giornate e Tabellini

1 GIORNATA

Sampdoria Femminile	0
Inter Women	2
Pomigliano Femminile	2
Juventus Women	3
Fiorentina Femminile	2
Sassuolo Femminile	1
Como Women	2
Napoli Femminile	1
Milan Femminile	2
Roma Femminile	4

Tabellini

17/09/2023 ore 18:00

SAMPDORIA FEMMINILE - INTER WOMEN 0-2

Reti: 12' Junge Pedersen (I), 18' Cambiaghi (I)

SAMPDORIA FEMMINILE (4-4-2): Karresmaa; De Rita, Oliviero, Heroum, Cuschier (71' Tatiely); Benoit, Schatzer, Bragonzi, Re; Giordano, Tarenzi

A disposizione: Tampieri, Marenco, Lazzeri, Grassi, Tonelli, Rosignoli

Allenatore: Salvatore Mango

INTER WOMEN (4-3-3): Cetinja; Thogersen (85' Merlo), Bowen, Tomter, Sonstevold; Karchouni, Junge Pedersen, Pandini; Bonfantini (78' Simonetti), Cambiaghi, Bugeja (65' Bonetti)

A disposizione: Piazza, Robustellini, Alborghetti, Eckhoff, Tironi, Jelcic

Allenatore: Rita Guarino

ARBITRO: Edoardo Gianquinto

AMMONITE: 57' Re (S)

ESPULSE: nessuna

16/09/2023 ore 15:00

POMIGLIANO FEMMINILE - JUVENTUS WOMEN 2-3

Reti: 11' Nambi (P), 29' Nilden (J), 31' Grosso (J), 33' Martinez Maldonado (P), 68' Girelli (J)

POMIGLIANO FEMMINILE (4-2-3-1): Gavillet; Novellino, Rabot, Caiazzo, Battistini; Di Giammarino (86' Talle), Ferrario; Nambi (78' Bourgoin), Ippolito (89' Manca), Martinez Maldonado; Szymanowski

A disposizione: Buhigas, Apicella, Fusini, Corrado, Domi, Tengue

Allenatore: Antonio Contreras

JUVENTUS WOMEN (4-3-3): Peyraud-Magnin; Lenzini (73' Gama), Sembrant, Cascarino, Nilden; Gunnarsdottir, Grosso, Palis (58' Caruso); Cantore, Nyström (58' Girelli), Beerensteyn (84' Thomas)

A disposizione: Aprile, Cocino, Cafferata, Bellucci, Moretti

Allenatore: Joseph Adrian Montemurro

ARBITRO: Gabriele Totaro

AMMONITE: 45' Cascarino (J); 63' Nilden (J)

ESPULSE: nessuna

16/09/2023 ore 18:00

FIORENTINA FEMMINILE - SASSUOLO FEMMINILE 2-1

Reti: 5' Sabatino (Rig.) (S), 8' Catena (F), 84' Cinotti (F)

FIORENTINA FEMMINILE (4-2-3-1): Schroffenegger; Faerge, Georgeva, Tortelli, Erzen (80' Toniolo); Severini (79' Cinotti), Breitner; Kajan (66' Longo), Boquete (88' Parisi), Catena; Mijatovic (88' Agard)

A disposizione: Baldi, Zanoli, Hammarlund, Lundin

Allenatore: Sebastian De La Fuente

SASSUOLO FEMMINILE (4-3-1-2): Durand; Orsi, Filangeri, Pleidrup, Philtjens; Mella (69' Santoro), Passeri (85' Ferrara), Brignoli (58' Prugna); Sciabica (46' Missipo); Sabatino, Beccari (68' Monterubbiano)

A disposizione: Kresche, Nagy, Tudisco, Brustia

Allenatore: Gianpiero Piovani

ARBITRO: Juan Luca Sacchi

AMMONITE: 45+3' Sciabica (S); 60' Mella (S); 64' Beccari (S)

ESPULSE: nessuna

17/09/2023 ore 12:30

COMO WOMEN - NAPOLI FEMMINILE 2-1

Reti: 31' Monnecchi (C), 59' Sevenius (C), 70' Del Estal (N)

COMO WOMEN (4-3-3): Korenciova; Lundorf Skovsen, Rizzon, Cox, Cecotti; Karlernas, Pastrenge (58' Hilaj), Vai-

tukaityt? (67' Picchi); Monnecchi (80' Lipman), Martinovic,
Arcangeli (57' Baldi)
A disposizione: Gilardi, Masu,
Bergersen Schaathun, Regaz-
zoli, Sevenius
Allenatore: Marco Bruzzano
NAPOLI FEMMINILE (4-3-
2-1): Bacic; Joy Friedichs (58'
Pettenuzzo), Di Marino, Di Bari
(65' Bertucci), Kobayashi; Co-
relli, Mauri, Banusic Meredinho
(58' Del Estal); Gallazzi, Chmie-
linski; Lazaro Torres Del Molino
A disposizione: Beretta, Fa-
biano, Veritti, Pellinghelli, Gia-
cobbo, Kajzba
Allenatore: Biagio Seno
ARBITRO: Silvia Gasperotti
AMMONITE: 9' Pastrenge (C);
14' Banusic Meredinho (N); 53'
Di Bari (N); 59' Gilardi (C)
ESPULSE: nessuna

17/09/2023 ore 15:00
**MILAN FEMMINILE - ROMA
FEMMINILE 2-4**
Reti: 36' Linari (R), 39' Haavi
(R), 50' Dompig (M), 61' Mari-
nelli (M), 80' Greggi (R), 90+3'
Glionna (R)
MILAN FEMMINILE (4-3-3):
Giuliani; Guagni, Arnadottir,
Swaby, Bergamaschi (68' Thri-
ge Andersen); Adami (75' Ma-
scarello), Cernoia, Grimshaw
(60' Marinelli); Laurent (75'
Asllani), Stašková, Dompig
A disposizione: Copetti, Fu-
setti, Soffia, Jonušait?, Arri-
goni
Allenatore: Maurizio Ganz
ROMA FEMMINILE (4-3-3):
Ceasar; Bartoli, Minami, Linari,
Di Guglielmo; Feiersinger (64'
Greggi), Giugliano, Kumagai;
Viens (64' Glionna), Giacinti
(89' Kramzar), Haavi (90+3'
Serturini)
A disposizione: Korpela, Val-
dezate, Aigbogun, Tomaselli,
Latorre
Allenatore: Alessandro Spu-
gna
ARBITRO: Domenico Castel-
lone
AMMONITE: nessuna
ESPULSE: nessuna

2

Roma Femminile	4
Como Women	1

Napoli Femminile	0
Milan Femminile	1

Sassuolo Femminile	1
Pomigliano Femminile	1

Juventus Women	4
Sampdoria Femminile	1

Inter Women	1
Fiorentina Femminile	1

Tabellini

30/09/2023 ore 15:00
**ROMA FEMMINILE - COMO
WOMEN 4-1**
Reti: 4' Kumagai (R), 56' Gia-
cinti (R), 88' Tomaselli (R), 90'
Martinovic (C), 90+3' Viens (R)
ROMA FEMMINILE (4-3-3):
Korpela; Bartoli, Valdezate,
Minami, Aigbogun; Latorre (59'
Glionna), Kumagai, Greggi (87'
Tomaselli); Giugliano (76' Fe-
iersinger), Giacinti (59' Viens),
Haavi (77' Serturini)
A disposizione: Ceasar, Di
Guglielmo, Ciccotti, Kramzar
Allenatore: Alessandro Spu-
gna
COMO WOMEN (4-3-3): Ko-
renciova; Lundorf Skovsen,
Rizzon, Cox (46' Lipman),
Cecotti; Karlernas, Hilaj (75'
Bergersen Schaathun), Vai-
tukaityt? (63' Regazzoli); Baldi
(57' Arcangeli), Sevenius (63'
Martinovic), Monnecchi
A disposizione: Gilardi, Masu,
Pastrenge, Picchi
Allenatore: Marco Bruzzano
ARBITRO: Gabriele Totaro
AMMONITE: 67' Lundorf
Skovsen (C); 84' Karlernas (C);

90+4' Regazzoli (C)
ESPULSE: nessuna

01/10/2023 ore 12:30
**NAPOLI FEMMINILE - MI-
LAN FEMMINILE 0-1**
Reti: 90+6' Laurent (M)
NAPOLI FEMMINILE (4-4-
2): Bacic; Pettenuzzo, Di Ma-
rino, Di Bari, Kobayashi; Joy
Friedichs (57' Giacobbo), Mauri
(81' Kajzba), Gallazzi, Chmie-
linski (69' Corelli); Banusic
Meredinho, Lazaro Torres Del
Molino (81' Del Estal)
A disposizione: Beretta, Fa-
biano, Veritti, Bertucci, Pellin-
ghelli
Allenatore: Biagio Seno
MILAN FEMMINILE (4-3-
3): Giuliani; Thrige Andersen
(67' Guagni), Arnadottir (77'
Swaby), Fusetti, Bergama-
schi; Grimshaw, Mascarel-
lo (59' Adami), Cernoia (77'
Jonušait?); Marinelli (67' Lau-
rent), Stašková, Dompig
A disposizione: Copetti, Piga,
Dubcová, Arrigoni
Allenatore: Maurizio Ganz
ARBITRO: Mauro Gangi
AMMONITE: 54' Pettenuzzo
(N); 73' Bacic (N); 90+5' Gallaz-
zi (N); 90+6' Marinelli (M)
ESPULSE: nessuna

01/10/2023 ore 14:30
**SASSUOLO FEMMINILE -
POMIGLIANO FEMMINILE
1-1**
Reti: 54' Harvey Lynn (P), 59'
Sabatino (S)
SASSUOLO FEMMINILE
(4-3-1-2): Durand; Orsi, Filan-
geri (80' Kullashi), Pleidrup,
Philtjens (63' Santoro); Missi-
po (46' Clelland), Pondini (62'
Brignoli), Passeri; Prugna; Sa-
batino, Beccari (74' Sciabica)
A disposizione: Kresche,
Nagy, Tudisco, Monterubbiano
Allenatore: Gianpiero Piovani
POMIGLIANO FEMMINILE
(4-4-2): Buhigas; Novellino
(80' Apicella), Rabot, Caiazzo,
Harvey Lynn; Szymanowski,
Ferrario (66' Bourgoin), Di
Giammarino, Ippolito (90+3'

Domi); Nambi (81' Battistini), Martinez Maldonado
A disposizione: Gavillet, Fusini, Corrado, Manca, Tengue
Allenatore: Antonio Contreras
ARBITRO: Gianluca Renzi
AMMONITE: 89' Battistini (P)
ESPULSE: nessuna

01/10/2023 ore 18:00
JUVENTUS WOMEN - SAMPDORIA FEMMINILE 4-1
Reti: 20' Garbino (J), 51' Tatiely (Rig.) (S), 63' Beerensteyn (J), 66' Girelli (J), 77' Beerensteyn (J)
JUVENTUS WOMEN (4-3-3): Peyraud-Magnin; Gama, Lenzini, Cascarino, Nilden; Gunnarsdottir, Garbino (75' Grosso), Caruso (83' Bellucci); Cantore (75' Thomas), Girelli (83' Nyström), Beerensteyn (78' Boattin)
A disposizione: Aprile, Salvai, Palis, Bonansea
Allenatore: Joseph Adrian Montemurro
SAMPDORIA FEMMINILE (4-4-2): Tampieri; De Rita, Heroum (74' Huchet), Pisani, Oliviero (79' Battelani); Giordano, Benoit, Re, Sondergaard (58' Cuschieri); Tatiely, Tarenzi (57' Bragonzi)
A disposizione: Karresmaa, Nespolo, Marenco, Schatzer, Grassi
Allenatore: Salvatore Mango
ARBITRO: Luca De Angeli
AMMONITE: 39' Tatiely (S); 43' Garbino (J); 50' Peyraud-Magnin (J); 56' Benoit (S); 56' Gunnarsdottir (J); 69' Gunnarsdottir (J); 90' Cascarino (J)
ESPULSE: 69' Gunnarsdottir (J)

02/10/2023 ore 18:00
INTER WOMEN - FIORENTINA FEMMINILE 1-1
Reti: 45+1' Mijatovic (F), 78' Junge Pedersen (I)
INTER WOMEN (4-3-3): Cetinja; Thogersen, Alborghetti, Bowen, Sonstevold; Simonetti, Junge Pedersen, Pandini (89'

Eckhoff); Nchout Njoya (56' Bonetti), Cambiaghi, Bugeja (63' Jelcic)
A disposizione: Piazza, Merlo, Robustellini, Tomter, Fadda, Tironi
Allenatore: Rita Guarino
FIORENTINA FEMMINILE (4-2-3-1): Schroffenegger; Faerge, Tortelli, Agard, Erzen; Severini (72' Hammarlund), Breitner; Catena (46' Cinotti), Boquete (71' Parisi), Mijatovic (81' Toniolo); Kajan (60' Longo)
A disposizione: Baldi, Spinelli, Zanoli, Lundin
Allenatore: Sebastian De La Fuente
ARBITRO: Andrea Calzavara
AMMONITE: 75' Schroffenegger (F); 85' Cambiaghi (I); 88' Parisi (F)
ESPULSE: nessuna

3

GIORNATA

| Sampdoria Femminile | 1 |
| Como Women | 2 |

| Pomigliano Femminile | 0 |
| Roma Femminile | 5 |

| Milan Femminile | 0 |
| Juventus Women | 1 |

| Fiorentina Femminile | 2 |
| Napoli Femminile | 0 |

| Sassuolo Femminile | 1 |
| Inter Women | 2 |

Tabellini

07/10/2023 ore 12:30
SAMPDORIA FEMMINILE - COMO WOMEN 1-2
Reti: 2' Karlernas (C), 15' Skorvankova (C), 76' Giordano (S)

SAMPDORIA FEMMINILE (4-3-3): Tampieri; De Rita, Heroum (57' Schatzer), Pisani, Oliviero; Giordano (90+1' Huchet), Benoit (87' Cuschieri), Re; Tarenzi (56' Sondergaard), Tatiely, Bragonzi (55' Battelani)
A disposizione: Karresmaa, Marenco, Lazzeri, Rosignoli
Allenatore: Salvatore Mango
COMO WOMEN (4-3-3): Korenciova; Cecotti, Rizzon, Cox, Lundorf Skovsen (82' Masu); Karlernas, Skorvankova (71' Regazzoli), Vaitukaityt? (61' Hilaj); Monnecchi (82' Martinovic), Sevenius, Arcangeli (60' Baldi)
A disposizione: Gilardi, Lipman, Pastrenge, Picchi
Allenatore: Marco Bruzzano
ARBITRO: Edoardo Manedo Mazzoni
AMMONITE: 38' De Rita (S); 49' Vaitukaityt? (C); 77' Sondergaard (S)
ESPULSE: nessuna

07/10/2023 ore 15:00
POMIGLIANO FEMMINILE - ROMA FEMMINILE 0-5
Reti: 9' Feiersinger (R), 20' Feiersinger (R), 44' Kumagai (R), 64' Viens (R), 90+4' Tomaselli (R)
POMIGLIANO FEMMINILE (4-4-2): Buhigas; Novellino (66' Battistini), Rabot, Caiazzo, Harvey Lynn; Szymanowski, Di Giammarino (90' Corrado), Bourgoin (73' Domi), Ippolito; Nambi (90' Manca), Martinez Maldonado
A disposizione: Gavillet, Apicella, Fusini, Ferrario, Tengue
Allenatore: Antonio Contreras
ROMA FEMMINILE (4-3-3): Ceasar; Aigbogun, Valdezate, Minami, Di Guglielmo; Feiersinger, Kumagai (74' Ciccotti), Giugliano (74' Tomaselli); Latorre (60' Serturini), Viens (74' Giacinti), Haavi (60' Kramzar)
A disposizione: Korpela, Bartoli, Greggi, Glionna
Allenatore: Alessandro Spu-

gna
ARBITRO: Antonio Di Reda
AMMONITE: 2' Di Guglielmo
(R); 36' Szymanowski (P); 82'
Valdezate (R)
ESPULSE: nessuna

07/10/2023 ore 19:00
**MILAN FEMMINILE - JU-
VENTUS WOMEN 0-1**
Reti: 87' Caruso (J)
MILAN FEMMINILE (4-3-3):
Giuliani; Guagni, Swaby, Fu-
setti, Bergamaschi; Grimshaw,
Cernoia (62' Mascarello), Dub-
cová (81' Adami); Laurent (72'
Marinelli), Stašková, Dompig
(82' Arnadottir)
A disposizione: Copetti, Thri-
ge Andersen, Piga, Asllani,
Arrigoni
Allenatore: Maurizio Ganz
JUVENTUS WOMEN (4-3-
3): Peyraud-Magnin; Boattin,
Lenzini, Cascarino, Nilden;
Caruso, Grosso, Garbino (64'
Bonansea); Cantore (46' Tho-
mas), Girelli (63' Nyström),
Beerensteyn (90+4' Bellucci)
A disposizione: Aprile, Salvai,
Sembrant, Cafferata, Palis
Allenatore: Joseph Adrian
Montemurro
ARBITRO: Alberto Ruben Are-
na
AMMONITE: 22' Garbino (J);
59' Cernoia (M); 85' Grimshaw
(M)
ESPULSE: nessuna

08/10/2023 ore 12:30
**FIORENTINA FEMMINILE -
NAPOLI FEMMINILE 2-0**
Reti: 83' Kajan (F), 86' Boque-
te (F)
FIORENTINA FEMMINILE
(4-3-3): Baldi; Erzen, George-
va, Tortelli, Faerge; Severini
(79' Parisi), Catena (79' To-
niolo), Breitner (70' Cinotti);
Mijatovic (60' Kajan), Boquete,
Hammarlund (61' Lundin)
A disposizione: Schroffeneg-
ger, Spinelli, Zanoli, Agard
Allenatore: Patrizia Panico
NAPOLI FEMMINILE (4-4-
2): Beretta; Pettenuzzo (88'
Bertucci), Di Marino, Di Bari,

Kobayashi; Joy Friedichs (57'
Giacobbo), Mauri, Gallazzi,
Chmielinski (46' Kajzba); Del
Estal (58' Banusic Meredinho),
Lazaro Torres Del Molino (66'
Corelli)
A disposizione: Fabiano, Ve-
ritti, Pellinghelli
Allenatore: Biagio Seno
ARBITRO: Luca Cherchi
AMMONITE: 22' Di Bari (N);
63' Georgeva (F); 69' Breitner
(F); 77' Giacobbo (N); 82' Pet-
tenuzzo (N)
ESPULSE: nessuna

08/10/2023 ore 15:00
**SASSUOLO FEMMINILE -
INTER WOMEN 1-2**
Reti: 53' Bonfantini (Rig.) (I),
75' Karchouni (I), 77' Nagy (S)
SASSUOLO FEMMINILE
(3-5-2): Kresche (22' Du-
rand); Orsi, Filangeri, Plei-
drup (62' Prugna); Santoro,
Brignoli, Pondini (70' Nagy),
Missipo (62' Monterubbiano),
Philtjens; Sabatino, Beccari
(63' Kullashi)
A disposizione: Mella, Tudi-
sco, Brustia, Sciabica
Allenatore: Gianpiero Piovani
INTER WOMEN (4-3-3): Ce-
tinja; Thogersen, Alborghetti,
Bowen, Sonstevold; Simonetti,
Junge Pedersen (33' Csiszár;
87' Polli), Karchouni; Bonfan-
tini (73' Merlo), Cambiaghi (72'
Nchout Njoya), Bugeja (46'
Bonetti)
A disposizione: Piazza, Robu-
stellini, Tomter, Fadda
Allenatore: Rita Guarino
ARBITRO: Simone Galipo
AMMONITE: 65' Karchouni (I);
67' Cetinja (I); 80' Simonetti (I);
82' Santoro (S); 89' Filangeri
(S)
ESPULSE: nessuna

4

Napoli Femminile	0
Sampdoria Femminile	2
Como Women	0
Milan Femminile	0
Pomigliano Femminile	1
Fiorentina Femminile	4
Roma Femminile	2
Inter Women	0
Juventus Women	4
Sassuolo Femminile	0

Tabellini

14/10/2023 ore 12:30
**NAPOLI FEMMINILE - SAM-
PDORIA FEMMINILE 0-2**
Reti: 6' De Rita (S), 19' Giorda-
no (S)
NAPOLI FEMMINILE (4-
3-3): Bacic; Pettenuzzo, Di
Marino, Di Bari (78' Bertucci),
Kobayashi; Giacobbo (46' Joy
Friedichs), Mauri (46' Kajzba),
Banusic Meredinho; Corelli,
Lazaro Torres Del Molino (46'
Gallazzi), Chmielinski
A disposizione: Veritti, Fa-
biano, Beretta, Del Estal, Pel-
linghelli
Allenatore: Biagio Seno
SAMPDORIA FEMMINILE
(4-4-2): Tampieri; De Rita (84'
Huchet), Pisani, Re, Oliviero;
Giordano (90+1' Sondergaard),
Schatzer, Benoit, Cuschieri;
Battelani (78' Heroum), Tatiely
A disposizione: Rosignoli,
Bragonzi, Tarenzi, Lazzeri,
Karresmaa, Marenco
Allenatore: Salvatore Mango
ARBITRO: Adolfo Baratta
AMMONITE: 25' Chmielinski
(N); 51' Corelli (N); 66' Di Bari
(N); 87' Re (S)

14/10/2023 ore 18:00

COMO WOMEN - MILAN FEMMINILE 0-0
COMO WOMEN (4-4-2): Korenciova; Lundorf Skovsen, Rizzon (65' Bergersen Schaathun), Cox, Cecotti; Monnecchi (78' Arcangeli), Hilaj (78' Pastrenge), Vaitukaityt? (57' Baldi), Skorvankova; Karlernas, Sevenius (79' Martinovic)
A disposizione: Gilardi, Lipman, Masu, Picchi
Allenatore: Marco Bruzzano
MILAN FEMMINILE (4-3-3): Giuliani; Arnadottir, Swaby, Piga, Bergamaschi; Dubcová (58' Asllani), Mascarello (76' Adami), Grimshaw; Laurent (82' Soffia), Stašková, Marinelli (58' Dompig)
A disposizione: Copetti, Thrige Andersen, Fusetti, Arrigoni, Aprile
Allenatore: Maurizio Ganz
ARBITRO: Abdoulaye Diop
AMMONITE: 8' Karlernas (C); 12' Mascarello (M); 18' Cecotti (C); 27' Piga (M); 32' Bergamaschi (M); 63' Hilaj (C)
ESPULSE: nessuna

15/10/2023 ore 12:30

POMIGLIANO FEMMINILE - FIORENTINA FEMMINILE 1-4
Reti: 18' Catena (F), 43' Boquete (F), 67' Longo (F), 78' Hammarlund (F), 90+1' Ippolito (Rig.) (P)
POMIGLIANO FEMMINILE (4-4-2): Buhigas; Novellino (87' Fusini), Rabot, Caiazzo, Harvey Lynn; Nambi, Di Giammarino (88' Domi), Ferrario (46' Apicella), Martinez Maldonado; Szymanowski (75' Bourgoin), Ippolito
A disposizione: Gavillet, Battistini, Corrado, Manca, Tengue
Allenatore: Antonio Contreras
FIORENTINA FEMMINILE (4-3-3): Baldi; Erzen (75' Agard), Georgeva, Tortelli, Faerge; Breitner (75' Parisi), Severini, Catena; Mijatovic (60' Longo), Lundin (60' Hammarlund), Boquete (81' Toniolo)
A disposizione: Schroffenegger, Spinelli, Zanoli, Kajan
Allenatore: Sebastian De La Fuente
ARBITRO: Dario Di Francesco
AMMONITE: 57' Ippolito (P); 57' Erzen (F)
ESPULSE: nessuna

15/10/2023 ore 16:00

ROMA FEMMINILE - INTER WOMEN 2-0
Reti: 18' Greggi (R), 66' Alborghetti (Aut.) (I)
ROMA FEMMINILE (4-3-3): Korpela; Aigbogun, Minami, Linari, Di Guglielmo; Giugliano, Kumagai, Greggi (83' Feiersinger); Glionna (59' Viens), Giacinti (69' Serturini), Haavi (83' Latorre)
A disposizione: Ceasar, Valdezate, Ciccotti, Tomaselli, Kramzar
Allenatore: Alessandro Spugna
INTER WOMEN (4-2-3-1): Cetinja; Sonstevold (86' Bonetti), Alborghetti, Bowen, Merlo; Csiszár (74' Bugeja), Eckhoff (46' Simonetti); Thogersen, Karchouni, Bonfantini; Cambiaghi (67' Nchout Njoya)
A disposizione: Piazza, Robustellini, Tomter, Fadda, Polli
Allenatore: Rita Guarino
ARBITRO: Marco Emmanuele
AMMONITE: 38' Aigbogun (R)
ESPULSE: nessuna

15/10/2023 ore 18:00

JUVENTUS WOMEN - SASSUOLO FEMMINILE 4-0
Reti: 6' Beerensteyn (J), 21' Girelli (J), 35' Beerensteyn (J), 45' Garbino (J)
JUVENTUS WOMEN (4-3-3): Peyraud-Magnin; Boattin, Lenzini, Cascarino (64' Salvai), Nilden; Grosso, Garbino (78' Palis), Caruso (78' Nyström); Bonansea (64' Gunnarsdottir), Girelli (79' Thomas), Beerensteyn
A disposizione: Gama, Toniolo, Bellucci, Aprile
Allenatore: Joseph Adrian Montemurro
SASSUOLO FEMMINILE (3-5-2): Durand; Passeri (60' Brignoli), Filangeri, Pleidrup; Santoro, Pondini (76' Brustia), Zamanian Le Loc'h Bakhtiari (68' Mella), Missipo, Philtjens; Monterubbiano (76' Sciabica), Sabatino (60' Kullashi)
A disposizione: Prugna, Nagy, Tudisco, Lonni
Allenatore: Gianpiero Piovani
ARBITRO: Giuseppe Vingo
AMMONITE: 26' Filangeri (S); 66' Peyraud-Magnin (J)
ESPULSE: 67' Santoro (S)

5

GIORNATA

Inter Women	2
Napoli Femminile	0
Sassuolo Femminile	1
Como Women	2
Milan Femminile	4
Pomigliano Femminile	1
Fiorentina Femminile	1
Juventus Women	2
Sampdoria Femminile	0
Roma Femminile	5

Tabellini

21/10/2023 ore 12:30

INTER WOMEN - NAPOLI FEMMINILE 2-0
Reti: 30' Simonetti (I), 46' Cambiaghi (I)
INTER WOMEN (4-3-3): Cetinja; Merlo, Tomter, Bowen, Sonstevold; Simonetti, Csiszár, Karchouni (68' Pandini); Bugeja (76' Nchout Njoya),

Cambiaghi (76' Polli), Bonfan-
tini (68' Bonetti)
A disposizione: Alborghetti,
Eckhoff, Thogersen, Piazza,
Robustellini
Allenatore: Rita Guarino
NAPOLI FEMMINILE (4-5-1):
Bacic; Kobayashi, Di Bari, Pel-
linghelli (62' Lazaro Torres Del
Molino), Veritti; Giacobbo (62'
Corelli), Mauri (70' Kajzba),
Chmielinski, Gallazzi (79' Del
Estal), Pettenuzzo (79' Bertuc-
ci); Banusic Meredinho
A disposizione: Di Marino,
Joy Friedichs, Fabiano, Beretta
Allenatore: Biagio Seno
ARBITRO: Antonino Costanza
AMMONITE: nessuna
ESPULSE: nessuna

21/10/2023 ore 18:00

**SASSUOLO FEMMINILE -
COMO WOMEN 1-2**
Reti: 19' Skorvankova (C), 67'
Zamanian Le Loc'h Bakhtiari
(S), 90+1' Orsi (Aut.) (S)
SASSUOLO FEMMINILE (3-
5-2): Kresche; Orsi, Filangeri,
Pleidrup; Brignoli, Pondini (74'
Ferrara), Zamanian Le Loc'h
Bakhtiari (89' Passeri), Missi-
po (46' Prugna), Philtjens; Sa-
batino, Clelland (55' Kullashi)
A disposizione: Durand, Mel-
la, Nagy, Sciabica, Monterub-
biano
Allenatore: Gianpiero Piovani
COMO WOMEN (4-3-3):
Korenciova; Cecotti, Berger-
sen Schaathun, Cox, Lundorf
Skovsen; Karlernas, Skor-
vankova (42' Hilaj), Vai-
tukaityt? (74' Picchi); Monnec-
chi (74' Arcangeli), Sevenius,
Martinovic (58' Baldi)
A disposizione: Gilardi,
Lipman, Masu, Pastrenge,
Bianchi
Allenatore: Marco Bruzzano
ARBITRO: Andrea Zoppi
AMMONITE: 80' Philtjens (S)
ESPULSE: nessuna

22/10/2023 ore 12:30

**MILAN FEMMINILE - POMI-
GLIANO FEMMINILE 4-1**
Reti: 2' Asllani (M), 29'
Stašková (M), 70' Martinez
Maldonado (P), 79' Asllani (M),
90+3' Grimshaw (Rig.) (M)
MILAN FEMMINILE (4-2-3-
1): Giuliani; Guagni (46' Soffia),
Swaby, Piga, Bergamaschi;
Grimshaw, Mascarello (86'
Adami); Laurent (46' Arna-
dottir), Asllani, Marinelli (46'
Dompig); Stašková (68' Vigi-
lucci)
A disposizione: Copetti, Fu-
setti, Cernoia, Jonušait?
Allenatore: Maurizio Ganz
POMIGLIANO FEMMINILE
(4-4-2): Buhigas; Novellino
(86' Fusini), Apicella, Corrado,
Harvey Lynn; Nambi, Rabot,
Di Giammarino (86' Domi),
Martinez Maldonado; Ippolito,
Szymanowski
A disposizione: Ferrario, Bat-
tistini, Gavillet, Caiazzo, Ten-
gue, Bourgoin, Manca
Allenatore: Antonio Contre-
ras
ARBITRO: Gabriele Sacchi
AMMONITE: 34' Di Giamma-
rino (P); 60' Novellino (P); 75'
Bergamaschi (M); 90+2' Buhi-
gas (P)
ESPULSE: nessuna

22/10/2023 ore 15:00

**FIORENTINA FEMMINILE -
JUVENTUS WOMEN 1-2**
Reti: 34' Beerensteyn (J), 67'
Catena (F), 77' Girelli (Rig.) (J)
**FIORENTINA FEMMINI-
LE** (4-3-3): Schroffenegger;
Tortelli, Georgeva, Erzen (82'
Toniolo), Faerge; Breitner (88'
Parisi), Severini (82' Agard),
Boquete; Mijatovic (62' Ham-
marlund), Longo (61' Catena),
Lundin
A disposizione: Baldi, Spinel-
li, Zanoli, Johannsdottir
Allenatore: Sebastian De La
Fuente
JUVENTUS WOMEN (4-3-3):
Peyraud-Magnin; Lenzini (74'
Gama), Salvai, Cascarino, Bo-
attin; Grosso, Caruso, Garbino
(87' Thomas); Beerensteyn,
Girelli (87' Nyström), Bonan-
sea (63' Gunnarsdottir)
A disposizione: Aprile, Tonio-

lo, Sembrant, Palis, Bellucci
Allenatore:
ARBITRO: Francesco Zago
AMMONITE: 39' Erzen (F); 41'
Grosso (J); 57' Georgeva (F);
60' Bonansea (J); 76' Georgeva
(F); 90+2' Nyström (J)
ESPULSE: 76' Georgeva (F)

22/10/2023 ore 17:00

**SAMPDORIA FEMMINILE -
ROMA FEMMINILE 0-5**
Reti: 45+2' Linari (R), 59' Viens
(R), 62' Giacinti (R), 66' Giacinti
(R), 90+1' Linari (Rig.) (R)
SAMPDORIA FEMMINILE
(4-3-2-1): Tampieri; De Ri-
ta, Benoit (67' Heroum), Re,
Oliviero; Giordano (90+1' Ro-
signoli), Huchet, Schatzer;
Battelani (87' Marenco), Cu-
schieri (67' Bragonzi); Tatiely
(87' Sondergaard)
A disposizione: Karresmaa,
Pisani, Lazzeri, Tarenzi
Allenatore: Salvatore Mango
ROMA FEMMINILE (4-3-3):
Ceasar; Bartoli, Minami, Linari,
Aigbogun (60' Di Guglielmo);
Giugliano (69' Tomaselli), Ku-
magai, Greggi (61' Feiersinger);
Viens, Giacinti (69' Kramzar),
Haavi (84' Latorre)
A disposizione: Korpela, Val-
dezate, Ciccotti, Glionna
Allenatore:
ARBITRO: Lorenzo Maccarini
AMMONITE: 24' Greggi (R);
44' Re (S); 62' Giacinti (R); 62'
Benoit (S); 86' Battelani (S);
90' Tampieri (S)
ESPULSE: nessuna

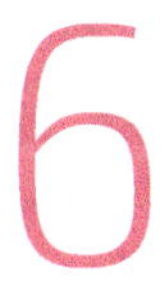

GIORNATA

Pomigliano Femminile	0
Sampdoria Femminile	1
Fiorentina Femminile	1
Milan Femminile	0

Juventus Women	1
Roma Femminile	3

Napoli Femminile	0
Sassuolo Femminile	1

Como Women	2
Inter Women	1

04/11/2023 ore 12:30

POMIGLIANO FEMMINILE - SAMPDORIA FEMMINILE 0-1

Reti: 82' Tatiely (Rig.) (S)
POMIGLIANO FEMMINILE (4-4-2): Buhigas; Harvey Lynn (84' Szymanowski), Apicella, Caiazzo, Fusini (90' Ferrario); Nambi (67' Novellino), Di Giammarino, Rabot, Martinez Maldonado; Ippolito, Bourgoin
A disposizione: Gavillet, Battistini, Corrado, Domi, Manca, Tengue
Allenatore: Antonio Contreras
SAMPDORIA FEMMINILE (4-3-3): Tampieri; De Rita, Pisani, Cuschieri (64' Huchet), Oliviero; Heroum, Benoit (64' Bragonzi), Schatzer; Re, Tatiely, Giordano (78' Battelani)
A disposizione: Karresmaa, Lindsay, Grassi, Sondergaard, Rosignoli, Tarenzi
Allenatore: Salvatore Mango
ARBITRO: Luigi Catanoso
AMMONITE: 27' Apicella (P); 45+1' Bourgoin (P); 50' Apicella (P); 67' Huchet (S); 71' Fusini (P); 74' Tatiely (S); 81' Harvey Lynn (P); 90+1' Bragonzi (S)
ESPULSE: 50' Apicella (P)

04/11/2023 ore 15:00

FIORENTINA FEMMINILE - MILAN FEMMINILE 1-0

Reti: 90+2' Mijatovic (F)
FIORENTINA FEMMINILE (4-2-3-1): Baldi; Erzen, Agard, Tortelli, Faerge (46' Toniolo); Severini (90+1' Johannsdottir), Breitner (76' Parisi); Catena, Boquete, Hammarlund (63' Mijatovic); Lundin (63' Longo)
A disposizione: Schroffenegger, Russo, Spinelli, Zanoli
Allenatore: Sebastian De La Fuente
MILAN FEMMINILE (4-2-3-1): Giuliani; Arnadottir, Swaby, Piga, Bergamaschi; Grimshaw (88' Adami), Cernoia (71' Asllani); Laurent (87' Soffia), Vigilucci, Dompig (46' Marinelli); Stašková
A disposizione: Babb, Fusetti, Guagni, Dubcová, Mascarello
Allenatore: Maurizio Ganz
ARBITRO: Michele Delrio
AMMONITE: 9' Dompig (M); 9' Severini (F); 75' Toniolo (F); 90+5' Adami (M)
ESPULSE: nessuna

05/11/2023 ore 12:30

JUVENTUS WOMEN - ROMA FEMMINILE 1-3

Reti: 27' Giugliano (R), 50' Haavi (R), 57' Viens (R), 60' Grosso (J)
JUVENTUS WOMEN (4-3-3): Peyraud-Magnin; Nilden (61' Gama), Salvai (79' Sembrant), Cascarino, Boattin; Grosso, Caruso, Garbino (61' Nyström); Bonansea (61' Cantore), Girelli, Beerensteyn
A disposizione: Aprile, Toniolo, Palis, Bellucci, Thomas
Allenatore: Joseph Adrian Montemurro
ROMA FEMMINILE (4-3-3): Ceasar; Di Guglielmo, Linari, Minami, Aigbogun; Greggi (73' Feiersinger), Kumagai, Giugliano (85' Tomaselli); Viens (62' Glionna), Giacinti (85' Kramzar), Haavi
A disposizione: Korpela, Valdezate, Ciccotti, Latorre, Pellegrino Cimo'
Allenatore: Alessandro Spugna
ARBITRO: Domenico Mirabella
AMMONITE: 12' Di Guglielmo (R); 22' Garbino (J); 41' Viens (R); 71' Aigbogun (R)
ESPULSE: nessuna

05/11/2023 ore 15:00

NAPOLI FEMMINILE - SASSUOLO FEMMINILE 0-1

Reti: 70' Sciabica (S)
NAPOLI FEMMINILE (4-3-3): Bacic; Pellinghelli (80' Bertucci), Di Marino (80' Pettenuzzo), Veritti, Kobayashi; Joy Friedichs (76' Corelli), Mauri, Kajzba (56' Gallazzi); Chmielinski (76' Del Estal), Lazaro Torres Del Molino, Banusic Meredinho
A disposizione: Beretta, Fabiano, Di Bari, Giacobbo
Allenatore: Biagio Seno
SASSUOLO FEMMINILE (4-3-3): Durand; Orsi, Filangeri, Pleidrup, Mella; Pondini (77' Prugna), Missipo, Brignoli (66' Santoro); Kullashi, Zamanian Le Loc'h Bakhtiari (66' Sciabica), Monterubbiano (66' Beccari)
A disposizione: Lonni, Philtjens, Tudisco, Sabatino, Clelland
Allenatore: Gianpiero Piovani
ARBITRO: Cristiano Ursini
AMMONITE: 35' Veritti (N); 72' Joy Friedichs (N); 78' Beccari (S)
ESPULSE: nessuna

05/11/2023 ore 18:00

COMO WOMEN - INTER WOMEN 2-1

Reti: 8' Picchi (C), 45' Bonfantini (Rig.) (I), 70' Sevenius (C)
COMO WOMEN (4-3-3): Korenciova; Lundorf Skovsen (84' Lipman), Rizzon, Cox, Cecotti; Hilaj (83' Pastrenge), Picchi (65' Karlernas), Vaitukaityt?; Baldi (75' Bergersen Schaathun), Sevenius, Monnecchi (83' Martinovic)
A disposizione: Gilardi, Masu, Bianchi, Arcangeli
Allenatore: Marco Bruzzano
INTER WOMEN (4-3-3): Cetinja; Merlo, Alborghetti, Bowen, Sonstevold; Simonetti, Csiszár, Karchouni (81' Bugeja); Bonetti (81' Jelcic), Cambiaghi (61' Polli), Bonfantini (89' Thogersen)
A disposizione: Durante, Robustellini, Tomter, Eckhoff,

Pandini
Allenatore: Rita Guarino
ARBITRO: Mattia Ubaldi
AMMONITE: 51' Karchouni (I); 90+2' Vaitukaityt? (C)
ESPULSE: nessuna

7

Como Women	0
Juventus Women	3

Sampdoria Femminile	0
Fiorentina Femminile	1

Inter Women	2
Pomigliano Femminile	1

Milan Femminile	1
Sassuolo Femminile	1

Roma Femminile	6
Napoli Femminile	0

Tabellini

12/11/2023 ore 20:30
COMO WOMEN - JUVENTUS WOMEN 0-3
Reti: 17' Salvai (J), 63' Caruso (J), 90+4' Thomas (J)
COMO WOMEN (4-3-3): Korenciova; Lundorf Skovsen (71' Skorvankova), Cox, Rizzon, Cecotti; Karlernas (79' Pastrenge), Hilaj (72' Arcangeli), Vaitukaityt?; Baldi (59' Bergersen Schaathun), Sevenius (79' Martinovic), Monnecchi
A disposizione: Gilardi, Lipman, Masu, Picchi
Allenatore: Marco Bruzzano
JUVENTUS WOMEN (4-3-3): Peyraud-Magnin; Lenzini (84' Gama), Salvai, Cascarino, Boattin (84' Nilden); Grosso, Caruso (75' Palis), Gunnarsdottir (51' Garbino); Cantore (75' Tho-

mas), Nyström, Beerensteyn
A disposizione: Aprile, Cafferata, Bellucci, Girelli
Allenatore: Joseph Adrian Montemurro
ARBITRO: Andrea Calzavara
AMMONITE: 81' Arcangeli (C)
ESPULSE: nessuna

12/11/2023 ore 12:30
SAMPDORIA FEMMINILE - FIORENTINA FEMMINILE 0-1
Reti: 86' Lundin (F)
SAMPDORIA FEMMINILE (4-3-3): Tampieri; De Rita, Giordano, Pisani, Oliviero (88' Sondergaard); Benoit, Schatzer (87' Tarenzi), Re; Huchet (65' Heroum), Tatiely (87' Battelani), Cuschieri (73' Bragonzi)
A disposizione: Karresmaa, Lindsay, Rosignoli
Allenatore: Salvatore Mango
FIORENTINA FEMMINILE (3-4-3): Schroffenegger; Erzen (64' Faerge), Tortelli, Agard (81' Georgeva); Catena, Severini, Breitner (46' Parisi), Toniolo (81' Johannsdottir); Mijatovic, Boquete, Longo (64' Lundin)
A disposizione: Zuluri, Baldi, Spinelli, Zanoli
Allenatore: Sebastian De La Fuente
ARBITRO: Maria Marotta
AMMONITE: 13' Giordano (S); 18' Mijatovic (F); 56' Huchet (S); 71' Catena (F); 74' Agard (F); 78' Parisi (F)
ESPULSE: nessuna

12/11/2023 ore 15:00
INTER WOMEN - POMIGLIANO FEMMINILE 2-1
Reti: 21' Ippolito (P), 36' Csiszár (I), 38' Bugeja (I)
INTER WOMEN (4-3-3): Cetinja; Thogersen, Tomter, Bowen, Robustellini (84' Sonstevold); Karchouni (83' Eckhoff), Csiszár, Pandini; Bonfantini, Cambiaghi, Bugeja (64' Polli)
A disposizione: Piazza, Durante, Alborghetti, Santi, Bonetti, Nchout Njoya

Allenatore: Rita Guarino
POMIGLIANO FEMMINILE (4-3-3): Buhigas; Battistini, Corrado, Caiazzo, Fusini; Di Giammarino (88' Domi), Rabot (75' Bourgoin), Ferrario (90+1' Manca); Nambi, Martinez Maldonado, Ippolito
A disposizione: Gavillet, Novellino, Schettino, Tengue
Allenatore: Alessandro Caruso
ARBITRO: Stefano Nicolini
AMMONITE: 25' Martinez Maldonado (P); 81' Karchouni (I); 88' Ippolito (P)
ESPULSE: nessuna

11/11/2023 ore 15:00
MILAN FEMMINILE - SASSUOLO FEMMINILE 1-1
Reti: 3' Bergamaschi (M), 6' Beccari (S)
MILAN FEMMINILE (4-2-3-1): Giuliani; Arnadottir (85' Soffia), Swaby, Thrige Andersen (71' Mascarello), Piga (54' Fusetti); Grimshaw, Vigilucci; Bergamaschi (85' Guagni), Asllani (71' Marinelli), Dompig; Stašková
A disposizione: Babb, Cernoia, Adami, Dubcová
Allenatore: Maurizio Ganz
SASSUOLO FEMMINILE (4-3-3): Durand; Orsi, Filangeri, Pleidrup, Santoro (86' Brignoli); Pondini, Missipo, Philtjens; Beccari (86' Sciabica), Zamanian Le Loc'h Bakhtiari, Clelland (71' Kullashi)
A disposizione: Kresche, Mella, Passeri, Nagy, Brustia, Sabatino
Allenatore: Gianpiero Piovani
ARBITRO: Carlo Rinaldi
AMMONITE: 45' Asllani (M); 66' Filangeri (S); 94' Durand (S)
ESPULSE: espulso l'allenatore Maurizio Ganz (Milan Femminile)

11/11/2023 ore 12:30
ROMA FEMMINILE - NAPOLI FEMMINILE 6-0
Reti: 19' Valdezate (R), 26' Di Guglielmo (R), 32' Viens (R), 45' Giugliano (R), 66' Di Gu-

glielmo (R), 90' Kramzar (R)
ROMA FEMMINILE (4-3-3): Korpela; Di Guglielmo, Valdezate, Linari (58' Minami), Aigbogun; Greggi, Kramzar, Giugliano (68' Feiersinger); Haavi (58' Latorre), Giacinti (68' Tomaselli), Viens (58' Glionna)
A disposizione: Ceasar, Kumagai, Ciccotti, Serturini
Allenatore: Alessandro Spugna
NAPOLI FEMMINILE (4-3-1-2): Beretta; Pellinghelli, Di Bari (61' Bertucci), Veritti, Corelli; Joy Friedichs (84' Kobayashi), Mauri (46' Giacobbo), Pettenuzzo; Chmielinski; Gallazzi, Del Estal (46' Banusic Meredinho)
A disposizione: Bacic, Cammarano, Di Marino
Allenatore: Biagio Seno
ARBITRO: Luca De Angeli
AMMONITE: 67' Corelli (N)
ESPULSE: nessuna

8

GIORNATA

Fiorentina Femminile	3
Como Women	0
Pomigliano Femminile	2
Napoli Femminile	1
Sassuolo Femminile	0
Roma Femminile	2
Juventus Women	5
Inter Women	0
Milan Femminile	1
Sampdoria Femminile	1

Tabellini

<u>18/11/2023 ore 15:00</u>
FIORENTINA FEMMINILE -

COMO WOMEN 3-0
Reti: 48' Boquete (Rig.) (F), 75' Longo (F), 78' Kajan (F)
FIORENTINA FEMMINILE (4-2-3-1): Baldi; Erzen, Georgeva, Tortelli, Faerge; Severini (83' Zanoli), Parisi (46' Johannsdottir); Lundin (63' Longo), Boquete (79' Breitner), Catena; Mijatovic (63' Kajan)
A disposizione: Schroffenegger, Spinelli, Toniolo, Agard
Allenatore: Sebastian De La Fuente
COMO WOMEN (4-3-3): Korenciova; Cecotti, Rizzon, Cox, Lundorf Skovsen (81' Bergersen Schaathun); Karlernas (46' Hilaj), Skorvankova (81' Picchi), Vaitukaityt? (81' Arcangeli); Baldi, Sevenius (72' Martinovic), Monnecchi
A disposizione: Gilardi, Lipman, Pastrenge, Di Luzio
Allenatore: Marco Bruzzano
ARBITRO: Fabrizio Pacella
AMMONITE: 84' Erzen (F); 85' Hilaj (C)
ESPULSE: nessuna

<u>19/11/2023 ore 18:00</u>
POMIGLIANO FEMMINILE - NAPOLI FEMMINILE 2-1
Reti: 27' Martinez Maldonado (P), 47' Giacobbo (N), 90+5' Rabot (Rig.) (P)
POMIGLIANO FEMMINILE (4-3-3): Buhigas; Battistini, Apicella, Caiazzo, Fusini; Di Giammarino (76' Domi), Rabot, Ferrario; Bourgoin (66' Nambi), Ippolito (89' Corrado), Martinez Maldonado
A disposizione: Gavillet, Harvey Lynn, Schettino, Szymanowski, Manca, Tengue
Allenatore: Alessandro Caruso
NAPOLI FEMMINILE (4-3-1-2): Bacic; Pettenuzzo, Joy Friedichs (46' Giacobbo), Veritti, Di Marino; Gallazzi, Mauri, Kobayashi; Chmielinski (82' Del Estal); Banusic Meredinho (67' Corelli), Lazaro Torres Del Molino
A disposizione: Beretta, Fabiano, Cammarano, Di Bari,

Bertucci, Pellinghelli
Allenatore: Biagio Seno
ARBITRO: Valerio Crezzini
AMMONITE: 38' Di Giammarino (P); 78' Mauri (N); 85' Rabot (P); 90+4' Lazaro Torres Del Molino (N)
ESPULSE: nessuna

<u>19/11/2023 ore 12:30</u>
SASSUOLO FEMMINILE - ROMA FEMMINILE 0-2
Reti: 15' Giugliano (R), 53' Kumagai (R)
SASSUOLO FEMMINILE (4-3-3): Durand; Orsi (61' Mella), Filangeri, Pleidrup, Philtjens; Pondini (74' Prugna), Missipo, Santoro; Beccari (71' Kullashi), Zamanian Le Loc'h Bakhtiari (46' Passeri), Clelland (61' Sabatino)
A disposizione: Kresche, Nagy, Brignoli, Sciabica
Allenatore: Gianpiero Piovani
ROMA FEMMINILE (4-3-3): Korpela; Bartoli, Minami, Linari, Aigbogun; Giugliano (74' Feiersinger), Kumagai (88' Ciccotti), Greggi; Haavi (66' Giacinti), Latorre (66' Glionna), Viens (74' Serturini)
A disposizione: Ceasar, Ohrstrom, Di Guglielmo, Tomaselli
Allenatore: Alessandro Spugna
ARBITRO: Gianluca Renzi
AMMONITE: nessuna
ESPULSE: nessuna

<u>19/11/2023 ore 16:00</u>
JUVENTUS WOMEN - INTER WOMEN 5-0
Reti: 2' Caruso (J), 5' Grosso (J), 52' Thomas (J), 60' Thomas (J), 79' Girelli (Rig.) (J)
JUVENTUS WOMEN (4-2-3-1): Peyraud-Magnin; Lenzini (74' Gama), Salvai, Cascarino, Boattin; Grosso (69' Palis), Caruso; Thomas, Garbino (74' Bellucci), Beerensteyn (69' Nilden); Nyström (74' Girelli)
A disposizione: Aprile, Sembrant, Cafferata, Cantore
Allenatore: Joseph Adrian Montemurro
INTER WOMEN (4-3-3):

Durante; Thogersen, Tomter, Bowen, Sonstevold (46' Robustellini); Pandini (51' Karchouni), Csiszár (90' Santi), Simonetti; Cambiaghi, Polli (74' Jelcic), Bonfantini (51' Bugeja)
A disposizione: Cetinja, Merlo, Alborghetti, Nchout Njoya
Allenatore: Rita Guarino
ARBITRO: Leonardo Mastrodomenico
AMMONITE: 90+2' Bellucci (J)
ESPULSE: nessuna

18/11/2023 ore 18:00
MILAN FEMMINILE - SAMPDORIA FEMMINILE 1-1
Reti: 7' Asllani (M), 70' Tatiely (Rig.) (S)
MILAN FEMMINILE (4-3-3): Giuliani; Arnadottir, Swaby, Piga, Guagni; Grimshaw (88' Stašková), Mascarello (63' Vigilucci), Cernoia (63' Adami); Bergamaschi (78' Laurent), Dompig, Asllani
A disposizione: Fusetti, Thrige Andersen, Marinelli, Soffia, Babb
Allenatore: Maurizio Ganz
SAMPDORIA FEMMINILE (4-5-1): Tampieri; De Rita, Re, Pisani, Oliviero; Giordano, Huchet, Benoit, Schatzer, Cuschieri (81' Heroum); Tatiely
A disposizione: Battelani, Karresmaa, Bragonzi, Rosignoli, Sondergaard, Lindsay, Tarenzi
Allenatore: Salvatore Mango
ARBITRO: Giuseppe Claudio Allegretta
AMMONITE: 14' Re (S); 47' Grimshaw (M); 69' Piga (M)
ESPULSE: nessuna

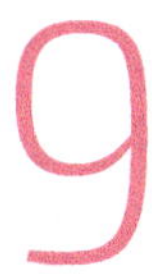

GIORNATA

Napoli Femminile	1
Juventus Women	3

Roma Femminile	2
Fiorentina Femminile	1

Sampdoria Femminile	0
Sassuolo Femminile	4

Inter Women	1
Milan Femminile	0

Como Women	0
Pomigliano Femminile	0

26/11/2023 ore 15:00
NAPOLI FEMMINILE - JUVENTUS WOMEN 1-3
Reti: 12' Gallazzi (N), 32' Caruso (J), 45' Caruso (Rig.) (J), 90+4' Thomas (J)
NAPOLI FEMMINILE (4-3-1-2): Bacic; Pettenuzzo, Di Marino, Di Bari, Pellinghelli; Giacobbo (80' Joy Friedichs), Mauri, Gallazzi; Chmielinski; Del Estal, Lazaro Torres Del Molino (76' Corelli)
A disposizione: Beretta, Fabiano, Cammarano, Kobayashi, Veritti, Bertucci, Banusic Meredinho
Allenatore: Biagio Seno
JUVENTUS WOMEN (4-3-3): Peyraud-Magnin; Lenzini, Salvai, Cascarino, Boattin; Grosso (8' Palis), Caruso, Thomas; Garbino, Beerensteyn, Nyström (67' Cantore)
A disposizione: Aprile, Gama, Nilden, Sembrant, Cafferata, Bellucci, Moretti
Allenatore:
ARBITRO: Samuele Andreano
AMMONITE: 45+3' Di Marino (N); 73' Caruso (J); 75' Del Estal (N); 90' Di Bari (N)
ESPULSE: nessuna

26/11/2023 ore 12:30
ROMA FEMMINILE - FIORENTINA FEMMINILE 2-1
Reti: 24' Greggi (R), 29' Longo (F), 60' Glionna (R)
ROMA FEMMINILE (4-3-3): Ceasar; Bartoli (63' Di Guglielmo), Minami, Linari, Aigbogun; Greggi (90+2' Valdezate), Kumagai, Giugliano; Glionna (64' Serturini), Giacinti (81' Feiersinger), Haavi
A disposizione: Korpela, Ciccotti, Tomaselli, Viens, Zouhir
Allenatore: Alessandro Spugna
FIORENTINA FEMMINILE (4-3-3): Baldi; Erzen (86' Agard), Georgeva, Tortelli, Faerge; Boquete, Johannsdottir (86' Toniolo), Severini (78' Parisi); Kajan (64' Mijatovic), Longo (64' Lundin), Catena
A disposizione: Schroffenegger, Russo, Zanoli, Mailia
Allenatore:
ARBITRO: Silvia Gasperotti
AMMONITE: 87' Serturini (R)
ESPULSE: nessuna

26/11/2023 ore 18:00
SAMPDORIA FEMMINILE - SASSUOLO FEMMINILE 0-4
Reti: 17' Kullashi (Sas), 42' Clelland (Sas), 46' Kullashi (Sas), 55' Kullashi (Sas)
SAMPDORIA FEMMINILE (4-3-3): Tampieri; De Rita (61' Battelani), Re, Pisani, Oliviero; Huchet (47' Heroum), Benoit, Cuschieri (47' Tarenzi); Giordano, Tatiely (77' Bragonzi), Schatzer
A disposizione: Karresmaa, Lindsay, Marenco, Sondergaard
Allenatore: Salvatore Mango
SASSUOLO FEMMINILE (4-3-3): Durand; Orsi, Filangeri, Pleidrup, Philtjens (83' Mella); Brignoli (62' Jane), Missipo, Pondini (77' Tudisco); Beccari, Kullashi (77' Zamanian Le Loc'h Bakhtiari), Clelland (77' Sabatino)
A disposizione: Lonni, Passeri, Santoro, Sciabica
Allenatore: Gianpiero Piovani
ARBITRO: Filippo Colaninno
AMMONITE: 16' Oliviero (Sam); 21' Brignoli (Sas)
ESPULSE: nessuna

25/11/2023 ore 13:45
INTER WOMEN - MILAN FEMMINILE 1-0

Reti: 72' Cambiaghi (I)
INTER WOMEN (4-3-3):
Durante; Thogersen, Tomter,
Bowen, Alborghetti; Simonetti,
Csiszár (74' Pandini), Karchou-
ni (90' Santi); Merlo, Cambia-
ghi, Polli (66' Jelcic)
A disposizione: Cetinja, Son-
stevold, Robustellini, Bugeja,
Bonfantini, Nchout Njoya
Allenatore: Rita Guarino
MILAN FEMMINILE (4-3-3):
Giuliani; Mascarello, Swaby,
Piga, Guagni (46' Arnadot-
tir); Grimshaw (83' Dubcová),
Stašková, Laurent (68' Viguluc-
ci); Bergamaschi, Dompig (82'
Marinelli), Asllani
A disposizione: Babb, Fusetti,
Soffia, Cernoia, Adami
Allenatore: Davide Corti
ARBITRO: Maria Marotta
AMMONITE: 30' Simonetti (I);
62' Karchouni (I); 67' Piga (M);
90+2' Asllani (M)
ESPULSE: nessuna

25/11/2023 ore 12:30
**COMO WOMEN - POMI-
GLIANO FEMMINILE 0-0**
COMO WOMEN (4-4-2): Ko-
renciova; Lundorf Skovsen (67'
Arcangeli), Rizzon, Cox, Cecot-
ti; Baldi (46' Bergersen Schaa-
thun), Pastrenge (57' Hilaj),
Vaitukaityt? (43' Karlernas),
Skorvankova; Monnecchi,
Martinovic (57' Sevenius)
A disposizione: Gilardi,
Lipman, Masu, Picchi
Allenatore: Marco Bruzzano
POMIGLIANO FEMMINILE
(4-4-2): Gavillet; Battistini,
Apicella, Caiazzo, Fusini; Bou-
rgoin (80' Ippolito), Ferrario
(84' Domi), Rabot, Di Giamma-
rino; Nambi (90+2' Corrado),
Martinez Maldonado
A disposizione: Buhigas,
Novellino, Schettino, Szyma-
nowski, Manca, Tengue
Allenatore: Alessandro Ca-
ruso
ARBITRO: Ermes Fabrizio Ca-
valiere
AMMONITE: 48' Skorvankova
(C); 65' Di Giammarino (P)
ESPULSE: nessuna

10

| Inter Women | 1 |
| Sampdoria Femminile | 1 |

| Napoli Femminile | 0 |
| Como Women | 0 |

| Roma Femminile | 2 |
| Milan Femminile | 1 |

| Sassuolo Femminile | 1 |
| Fiorentina Femminile | 2 |

| Juventus Women | 4 |
| Pomigliano Femminile | 0 |

Tabellini

09/12/2023 ore 12:30
**INTER WOMEN - SAMPDO-
RIA FEMMINILE 1-1**
Reti: 6' Schatzer (S), 78' Bon-
fantini (I)
INTER WOMEN (3-5-2):
Cetinja; Bowen, Alborghetti,
Tomter (75' Jelcic); Sonste-
vold, Csiszár, Karchouni, Si-
monetti (75' Nchout Njoya),
Robustellini (64' Thogersen);
Cambiaghi, Polli (46' Bonfan-
tini)
A disposizione: Piazza, Belli,
Santi, Pandini, Bugeja
Allenatore: Rita Guarino
SAMPDORIA FEMMINILE
(4-3-3): Tampieri; Heroum, Re,
De Rita, Oliviero; Giordano (90'
Battelani), Benoit, Schatzer;
Cuschieri (81' Pisani), Tatiely,
Sondergaard (72' Bragonzi)
A disposizione: Karresmaa,
Lindsay, Marenco, Huchet,
Tarenzi
Allenatore: Salvatore Mango
ARBITRO: Aleksandar
Djurdjevic
AMMONITE: 25' Cuschieri (S);
26' Alborghetti (I); 45' Simo-
netti (I); 66' Bonfantini (I)

ESPULSE: nessuna

10/12/2023 ore 15:00
**NAPOLI FEMMINILE - CO-
MO WOMEN 0-0**
NAPOLI FEMMINILE (4-3-1-
2): Bacic; Bertucci, Pettenuzzo,
Di Bari, Kobayashi; Giacobbo
(73' Joy Friedichs), Mauri, Gal-
lazzi; Chmielinski (72' Banusic
Meredinho); Del Estal, Lazaro
Torres Del Molino
A disposizione: Beretta, Fa-
biano, Cammarano, Veritti,
Pellinghelli
Allenatore: Biagio Seno
COMO WOMEN (4-2-3-1):
Korenciova; Cecotti, Rizzon,
Cox, Lundorf Skovsen; Karler-
nas, Hilaj (72' Arcangeli); Mon-
necchi (81' Di Luzio), Picchi,
Skorvankova; Sevenius (72'
Baldi)
A disposizione: Gilardi,
Lipman, Masu, Pastrenge, Ber-
gersen Schaathun, Martinovic
Allenatore: Marco Bruzzano
ARBITRO: Simone Galipo
AMMONITE: 8' Cox (C); 37' Gia-
cobbo (N); 44' Pettenuzzo (N)
ESPULSE: nessuna

10/12/2023 ore 12:30
**ROMA FEMMINILE - MILAN
FEMMINILE 2-1**
Reti: 24' Asllani (Rig.) (M), 58'
Giugliano (R), 64' Di Guglielmo
(R)
ROMA FEMMINILE (4-3-3):
Ceasar; Di Guglielmo, Minami,
Linari, Aigbogun; Giugliano
(90+3' Tomaselli), Kumagai,
Greggi; Glionna (69' Serturini),
Giacinti, Haavi
A disposizione: Korpela,
Ohrstrom, Valdezate, Ciccotti,
Feiersinger, Pellegrino Cimo',
Zouhir
Allenatore: Alessandro Spu-
gna
MILAN FEMMINILE (4-3-3):
Giuliani; Guagni (64' Arnadot-
tir), Swaby, Piga, Bergamaschi;
Grimshaw (86' Adami), Cerno-
ia (86' Vigilucci), Dubcová (69'
Marinelli); Laurent, Stašková
(64' Dompig), Asllani
A disposizione: Babb, Fusetti,

Soffia, Mascarello
Allenatore: Davide Corti
ARBITRO: Filippo Giaccaglia
AMMONITE: 27' Di Guglielmo (R); 32' Bergamaschi (M); 57' Grimshaw (M); 90' Giacinti (R)
ESPULSE: nessuna

11/12/2023 ore 18:00
SASSUOLO FEMMINILE - FIORENTINA FEMMINILE 1-2
Reti: 52' Catena (F), 73' Catena (F), 85' Beccari (S)
SASSUOLO FEMMINILE (4-3-3): Durand; Orsi, Filangeri, Pleidrup, Philtjens (87' Monterubbiano); Pondini (80' Brignoli), Missipo, Jane (65' Sabatino); Beccari, Kullashi (80' Santoro), Clelland
A disposizione: Kresche, Mella, Passeri, Prugna, Sciabica
Allenatore: Gianpiero Piovani
FIORENTINA FEMMINILE (4-3-3): Schroffenegger; Erzen (84' Zanoli), Georgeva, Agard, Faerge; Severini, Parisi (77' Johannsdottir), Catena; Mijatovic (63' Kajan), Longo (63' Hammarlund), Boquete (77' Spinelli)
A disposizione: Baldi, Russo, Toniolo, Lundin
Allenatore: Sebastian De La Fuente
ARBITRO: Gabriele Sacchi
AMMONITE: 34' Boquete (F); 37' Pleidrup (S); 71' Filangeri (S); 90+1' Severini (F)
ESPULSE: nessuna

09/12/2023 ore 15:00
JUVENTUS WOMEN - POMIGLIANO FEMMINILE 4-0
Reti: 30' Gunnarsdottir (J), 66' Beerensteyn (J), 70' Beerensteyn (J), 90+4' Bonansea (Rig.) (J)
JUVENTUS WOMEN (4-3-3): Aprile; Lenzini, Salvai (75' Cafferata), Cascarino, Boattin (84' Nilden); Caruso (83' Bellucci), Gunnarsdottir (83' Garbino), Palis; Thomas, Cantore (75' Bonansea), Beerensteyn
A disposizione: Peyraud-

Magnin, Sliskovic, Sembrant, Bellagente
Allenatore: Joseph Adrian Montemurro
POMIGLIANO FEMMINILE (4-3-1-2): Gavillet; Battistini, Apicella, Caiazzo, Fusini (85' Manca); Rabot, Ferrario, Di Giammarino (85' Tengue); Ippolito (85' Domi); Bourgoin (64' Nambi), Martinez Maldonado (74' Harvey Lynn)
A disposizione: Buhigas, Corrado, Novellino, Schettino
Allenatore:
ARBITRO: Mattia Caldera
AMMONITE: nessuna
ESPULSE: nessuna

11

Sampdoria Femminile	1
Juventus Women	0
Pomigliano Femminile	0
Sassuolo Femminile	2
Milan Femminile	1
Napoli Femminile	1
Fiorentina Femminile	4
Inter Women	2
Como Women	2
Roma Femminile	3

Tabellini

16/12/2023 ore 14:30
SAMPDORIA FEMMINILE - JUVENTUS WOMEN 1-0
Reti: 81' Bragonzi (S)
SAMPDORIA FEMMINILE (4-3-3): Tampieri; Heroum, Re, De Rita, Oliviero; Giordano, Benoit, Schatzer; Pisani, Tatiely, Tarenzi (70' Bragonzi)
A disposizione: Karresmaa,

Lindsay, Marenco, Cuschieri, Grassi, Battelani, Sondergaard, Rosignoli
Allenatore: Stefano Castiglione
JUVENTUS WOMEN (4-3-3): Peyraud-Magnin; Cafferata (60' Nilden), Salvai, Cascarino, Boattin; Caruso, Gunnarsdottir, Palis (66' Garbino); Thomas, Cantore (66' Bonansea), Beerensteyn
A disposizione: Aprile, Sembrant, Sliskovic, Lenzini, Bellucci, Moretti
Allenatore: Joseph Adrian Montemurro
ARBITRO: Giorgio Bozzetto
AMMONITE: 29' Benoit (S); 61' De Rita (S); 87' Salvai (J)
ESPULSE: nessuna

17/12/2023 ore 12:30
POMIGLIANO FEMMINILE - SASSUOLO FEMMINILE 0-2
Reti: 4' Kullashi (S), 48' Clelland (S)
POMIGLIANO FEMMINILE (4-3-1-2): Buhigas; Harvey Lynn, Caiazzo, Apicella, Fusini (83' Battistini); Di Giammarino (71' Novellino), Ferrario, Rabot; Ippolito; Bourgoin (83' Manca), Nambi (59' Martinez Maldonado)
A disposizione: Gavillet, Corrado, Schettino, Domi, Tengue
Allenatore: Alessandro Caruso
SASSUOLO FEMMINILE (4-3-3): Durand; Orsi, Filangeri, Pleidrup, Mella (59' Philtjens); Jane (46' Prugna), Missipo, Brignoli; Clelland (79' Sabatino), Kullashi (69' Santoro), Beccari (79' Monterubbiano)
A disposizione: Kresche, Passeri, Tudisco, Sciabica
Allenatore: Gianpiero Piovani
ARBITRO: Valerio Vogliacco
AMMONITE: 38' Nambi (P); 53' Mella (S); 78' Beccari (S)
ESPULSE: nessuna

16/12/2023 ore 12:30
MILAN FEMMINILE - NAPOLI FEMMINILE 1-1
Reti: 58' Del Estal (N), 90+6'

Laurent (M)

MILAN FEMMINILE (4-2-3-1): Babb; Bergamaschi, Swaby, Piga (73' Fusetti), Thrige Andersen (73' Soffia); Grimshaw, Rubio Avila (65' Vigilucci); Laurent, Asllani (64' Mascarello), Dompig; Stašková (40' Marinelli)

A disposizione: Giuliani, Cernoia, Adami, Arrigoni

Allenatore: Davide Corti

NAPOLI FEMMINILE (4-3-1-2): Bacic; Bertucci, Pettenuzzo, Di Bari, Kobayashi; Giacobbo (85' Pellinghelli), Mauri, Gallazzi; Chmielinski (79' Veritti); Lazaro Torres Del Molino (83' Banusic Meredinho), Del Estal

A disposizione: Beretta, Fabiano, Cammarano, D'Angelo, Langella

Allenatore: Biagio Seno

ARBITRO: Giuseppe Maria Manzo

AMMONITE: 53' Kobayashi (N); 69' Mascarello (M); 74' Bertucci (N); 80' Vigilucci (M); 90+3' Bacic (N)

ESPULSE: nessuna

18/12/2023 ore 18:00

FIORENTINA FEMMINILE - INTER WOMEN 4-2

Reti: 2' Cambiaghi (I), 50' Boquete (F), 56' Boquete (Rig.) (F), 58' Cambiaghi (I), 80' Boquete (F), 90' Catena (F)

FIORENTINA FEMMINILE (4-3-3): Baldi; Erzen (87' Spinelli), Georgeva, Agard, Faerge; Severini, Parisi (69' Johannsdottir), Catena; Mijatovic (75' Toniolo), Lundin (69' Longo), Boquete (88' Hammarlund)

A disposizione: Schroffenegger, Zanoli, Cinotti, Kajan

Allenatore: Sebastian De La Fuente

INTER WOMEN (3-5-2): Cetinja; Bowen, Alborghetti (86' Jelcic), Tomter; Thogersen, Karchouni (14' Pandini), Csiszár (78' Santi), Simonetti (85' Bugeja), Merlo; Cambiaghi, Bonfantini (78' Polli)

A disposizione: Piazza, Son-

stevold, Robustellini, Nchout Njoya

Allenatore: Rita Guarino

ARBITRO: Gabriele Scatena

AMMONITE: 45+3' Parisi (F); 55' Alborghetti (I); 90+4' Longo (F)

ESPULSE: nessuna

17/12/2023 ore 15:00

COMO WOMEN - ROMA FEMMINILE 2-3

Reti: 35' Skorvankova (C), 53' Linari (Rig.) (R), 56' Picchi (C), 59' Di Guglielmo (R), 62' Linari (Rig.) (R)

COMO WOMEN (4-4-2): Korenciova; Bergersen Schaathun, Rizzon, Cox, Lundorf Skovsen; Monnecchi, Karlernas, Vaitukaityt? (57' Hilaj), Picchi (78' Martinovic); Arcangeli (63' Baldi), Skorvankova

A disposizione: Gilardi, Lipman, Masu, Pastrenge, Bianchi, Di Luzio

Allenatore: Marco Bruzzano

ROMA FEMMINILE (4-3-3): Korpela; Bartoli, Valdezate, Linari, Di Guglielmo (78' Serturini); Tomaselli (46' Kumagai), Giugliano, Greggi (68' Feiersinger); Glionna (46' Giacinti), Viens, Haavi (68' Aigbogun)

A disposizione: Ceasar, Minami, Ciccotti, Pellegrino Cimo'

Allenatore: Alessandro Spugna

ARBITRO: Mattia Nigro

AMMONITE: 45+3' Skorvankova (C); 59' Hilaj (C)

ESPULSE: nessuna

12

Como Women	0
Sampdoria Femminile	1
Napoli Femminile	2
Fiorentina Femminile	4

Juventus Women	2
Milan Femminile	1
Inter Women	0
Sassuolo Femminile	1
Roma Femminile	3
Pomigliano Femminile	0

14/01/2024 ore 15:00

COMO WOMEN - SAMPDORIA FEMMINILE 0-1

Reti: 8' Schatzer (S)

COMO WOMEN (4-4-2): Korenciova; Bergersen Schaathun (79' Lundorf Skovsen), Rizzon, Cox, Cecotti; Monnecchi (46' Martinovic), Karlernas Hilaj (74' Lipman), Picchi (63' Vaitukaityte); Sevenius (74' Arcangeli), Skorvankova

A disposizione: Gilardi, Liva, Pastrenge, Bianchi

Allenatore: Marco Bruzzano

SAMPDORIA FEMMINILE (4-4-2): Tampieri; De Rita, Pisani, Re, Oliviero; Heroum (74' Nagy), Benoit, Schatzer, Cuschieri (89' Della Peruta V.); Battelani (82' Fallico), Tatiely

A disposizione: Karresmaa, Marenco, Micheli, Della Peruta T., Sondergaard, Tarenzi

Allenatore: Salvatore Mango

ARBITRO: Enrico Cappai

AMMONITE: 50' De Rita (S)

ESPULSE: nessuno

13/01/2024 ore 12:30

NAPOLI FEMMINILE - FIORENTINA FEMMINILE 2-4

Reti: 32' Boquete (F), 57' Catena (F), 72' Del Estal (Rig.) (N), 73' Longo (F), 80' Corelli (N), 87' Johannsdottir (F)

NAPOLI FEMMINILE (4-3-1-2): Bacic; Bertucci, Pettenuzzo, Di Bari, Kobayashi; Giacobbo, Gallazzi, Pellinghelli (59' Kajzba); Chmielinski; Lazaro Torres Del Molino (53' Corelli), Del Estal

A disposizione: Fabiano, Mauri, Beretta, Di Marino,

Langella, Banusic Meredinho, Cammarano
Allenatore: Biagio Seno
FIORENTINA FEMMINI-LE (4-3-3): Schroffenegger; Erzen (76' Toniolo), Agard, Georgeva, Faerge; Parisi (77' Johannsdottir), Severini, Catena; Boquete (84' Spinelli), Lundin (64' Longo), Mijatovic (64' Janogy)
A disposizione: Cinotti, Baldi, Zanoli, Hammarlund
Allenatore: Sebastian De La Fuente
ARBITRO: Erminio Cerbasi
AMMONITE: 90+1' Gallazzi (N)
ESPULSE: nessuna

13/01/2024 ore 16:15
JUVENTUS WOMEN - MILAN FEMMINILE 2-1
Reti: 25' Bonansea (J), 31' Stašková (M), 52' Cantore (J)
JUVENTUS WOMEN (4-3-3): Peyraud-Magnin; Lenzini, Salvai, Cascarino, Boattin; Garbino (88' Echegini), Gunnarsdottir, Caruso; Cantore, Bonansea, Thomas (74' Girelli)
A disposizione: Aprile, Gama, Sliskovic, Cafferata, Grosso, Bellucci, Bragonzi
Allenatore: Joseph Adrian Montemurro
MILAN FEMMINILE (4-3-3): Giuliani; Guagni, Swaby, Piga, Bergamaschi; Vigilucci (84' Rubio Avila), Cernoia, Grimshaw; Laurent, Stašková (63' Dompig), Asllani
A disposizione: Babb, Fusetti, Soffia, Dubcová, Mascarello, Arrigoni, Marinelli
Allenatore: Davide Corti
ARBITRO: Lorenzo Maccarini
AMMONITE: 61' Cernoia (M); 76' Laurent (M); 79' Lenzini (J)
ESPULSE: nessuna

14/01/2024 ore 12:30
INTER WOMEN - SASSUO-LO FEMMINILE 0-1
Reti: 27' Beccari (S)
INTER WOMEN (3-5-2): Cetinja; Tomter, Alborghetti, Bowen; Thogersen (73' Robustel-

lini), Simonetti (67' Bugeja), Csiszár, Pandini (46' Junge Pedersen), Merlo; Bonfantini (46' Jelcic), Cambiaghi
A disposizione: Polli, Santi, Belli, Nchout Njoya, Piazza
Allenatore: Rita Guarino
SASSUOLO FEMMINILE (4-3-3): Durand; Orsi, Filangeri, Pleidrup, Philtjens; Prugna (77' Santoro), Missipo, Brignoli (71' Pondini); Sabatino, Kullashi (85' Tudisco), Beccari
A disposizione: Mella, Lonni, Passeri, Mihelic, Sciabica, Monterubbiano
Allenatore: Gianpiero Piovani
ARBITRO: Marco Peletti
AMMONITE: 87' Csiszár (I)
ESPULSE: nessuna

13/01/2024 ore 18:00
ROMA FEMMINILE - POMI-GLIANO FEMMINILE 3-0
Reti: 12' Viens (R), 29' Feiersinger (R), 52' Haavi (R)
ROMA FEMMINILE (4-3-3): Ceasar; Di Guglielmo (76' Glionna), Bartoli, Linari, Minami; Feiersinger, Kumagai (82' Ciccotti), Giugliano (76' Greggi); Viens (63'), Giacinti, Haavi (63' Latorre)
A disposizione: Korpela, Valdezate, Tomaselli, Serturini, Pellegrino Cimo'
Allenatore: Alessandro Spugna
POMIGLIANO FEMMINILE (4-4-1-1): Gavillet; Harvey Lynn (90+2' Vingiani), Caiazzo, Apicella, Fusini; Novellino, Rabot (78' Domi), Ferrario (58' Szymanowski), Di Giammarino; Ippolito (90'); Nambi (79' Manca)
A disposizione: Buhigas, Battistini, Schettino
Allenatore: Alessandro Caruso
ARBITRO: Jules Roland Andeng Tona Mbei
AMMONITE: nessuna
ESPULSE: nessuna

13

Sampdoria Femminile	0
Napoli Femminile	0
Inter Women	2
Roma Femminile	0
Sassuolo Femminile	0
Juventus Women	1
Milan Femminile	3
Como Women	2
Fiorentina Femminile	3
Pomigliano Femminile	1

Tabellini

20/01/2024 ore 12:30
SAMPDORIA FEMMINILE - NAPOLI FEMMINILE 0-0
SAMPDORIA FEMMINILE (4-4-2): Tampieri; De Rita, Pisani, Re, Oliviero; Heroum (70' Tarenzi), Benoit, Schatzer, Cuschieri (81' Giordano); Battelani (70' Fallico), Tatiely
A disposizione: Karresmaa, Marenco, Nagy, Brustia, Della Peruta V., Sondergaard
Allenatore: Stefano Castiglione
NAPOLI FEMMINILE (4-3-1-2): Bacic; Pettenuzzo, Di Marino, Di Bari (90' Bertucci), Kobayashi; Giai (89' Kajzba), Gallazzi, Pellinghelli; Chmielinski; Del Estal, Corelli (78' Banusic Meredinho)
A disposizione: Beretta, Fabiano, Veritti, Giacobbo, Mauri, Lazaro Torres Del Molino
Allenatore: Biagio Seno
ARBITRO: Emanuele Ceriello
AMMONITE: 18' Re (S); 59' Corelli (N); 75' Di Bari (N); 75' Tatiely (S)
ESPULSE: nessuno

INTER WOMEN - ROMA FEMMINILE 2-0
Reti: 31' Bonfantini (I), 89' Polli (I)
INTER WOMEN (3-5-2): Cetinja; Tomter, Alborghetti, Bowen; Thogersen, Magull, Junge Pedersen, Santi, Merlo (69' Robustellini); Bonfantini (64' Polli), Cambiaghi (85' Jelcic)
A disposizione: Piazza, Pandini, Simonetti, Fadda, Bugeja, Tironi
Allenatore: Rita Guarino
ROMA FEMMINILE (4-3-3): Ceasar; Di Guglielmo (75' Feiersinger), Linari, Minami, Sonstevold; Greggi (75' Glionna), Kumagai, Giugliano; Viens, Giacinti (71' Latorre), Haavi
A disposizione: Korpela, Valdezate, Bartoli, Testa, Ciccotti, Pellegrino Cimo'
Allenatore: Alessandro Spugna
ARBITRO: Samuele Andreano
AMMONITE: 90+4' Polli (I)
ESPULSE: 63' Bartoli (R)

SASSUOLO FEMMINILE - JUVENTUS WOMEN 0-1
Reti: 89' Echegini (J)
SASSUOLO FEMMINILE (4-3-1-2): Durand; Orsi, Filangeri, Pleidrup, Philtjens; Pondini (75' Mihelic), Missipo, Brignoli (58' Kullashi); Prugna; Sabatino, Beccari (69' Clelland)
A disposizione: Lonni, Mella, Passeri, Santoro, Sciabica, Monterubbiano
Allenatore: Gianpiero Piovani
JUVENTUS WOMEN (4-3-3): Peyraud-Magnin; Lenzini (90+7' Gama), Calligaris, Cascarino, Boattin; Garbino (66' Girelli), Grosso, Caruso; Beerensteyn, Bonansea (90+7' Thomas), Cantore (78' Echegini)
A disposizione: Aprile, Salvai, Palis, Bellucci, Bragonzi
Allenatore: Joseph Adrian Montemurro
ARBITRO: Andrea Ancora
AMMONITE: 82' Mihelic (S)

ESPULSE: nessuna

MILAN FEMMINILE - COMO WOMEN 3-2
Reti: 12' Stašková (M), 43' Mascarello (M), 62' Stašková (M), 79' Skorvankova (C), 90+4' Martinovic (C)
MILAN FEMMINILE (4-3-3): Giuliani; Guagni, Swaby, Piga, Soffia; Dubcová, Mascarello (75' Vigilucci), Grimshaw (87' Mesjasz); Asllani (75' Rubio Avila), Stašková (87' Marinelli), Laurent (70' Dompig)
A disposizione: Copetti, Fusetti, Cesarini, Arrigoni
Allenatore: Davide Corti
COMO WOMEN (4-4-2): Korenciova; Lundorf Skovsen (46' Bergersen Schaathun), Rizzon, Cox, Cecotti; Picchi (46' Karlernas), Hilaj (69' Pastrenge), Vaitukaityt? (80' Colombo), Monnecchi (69' Martinovic); Sevenius, Skorvankova
A disposizione: Gilardi, Lipman, Bianchi, Arcangeli
Allenatore: Marco Bruzzano
ARBITRO: Davide Gandino
AMMONITE: 37' Picchi (C); 63' Hilaj (C); 90' Rizzon (C); 90' Mesjasz (M)
ESPULSE: nessuna

FIORENTINA FEMMINILE - POMIGLIANO FEMMINILE 3-1
Reti: 23' Johannsdottir (F), 41' Ferrario (P), 77' Janogy (F), 82' Janogy (F)
FIORENTINA FEMMINILE (4-3-3): Schroffenegger; Erzen (74' Hammarlund), Toniolo (74' Faerge), Georgeva, Spinelli; Johannsdottir, Severini, Catena (85' Agard); Boquete, Longo (60' Lundin), Mijatovic (60' Janogy)
A disposizione: Baldi, Tortelli, Zanoli, Cinotti
Allenatore: Sebastian De La Fuente
POMIGLIANO FEMMINILE (4-4-2): Buhigas; Harvey Lynn, Caiazzo, Apicella, Fusini

(83' Battistini); Novellino (83' Szymanowski), Rabot, Ferrario, Di Giammarino (83' Domi); Ippolito, Nambi (87' Manca)
A disposizione: Gavillet, Vingiani, Schettino
Allenatore: Alessandro Caruso
ARBITRO: Simone Gavini
AMMONITE: 57' Di Giammarino (P); 66' Buhigas (P); 75' Ippolito (P)
ESPULSE: nessuna

14
GIORNATA

Juventus Women	2
Fiorentina Femminile	2
Roma Femminile	2
Sampdoria Femminile	0
Pomigliano Femminile	0
Milan Femminile	0
Como Women	0
Sassuolo Femminile	1
Napoli Femminile	2
Inter Women	3

Tabellini

JUVENTUS WOMEN - FIORENTINA FEMMINILE 2-2
Reti: 19' Janogy (F), 26' Grosso (J), 32' Janogy (F), 74' Echegini (J)
JUVENTUS WOMEN (4-3-3): Peyraud-Magnin; Lenzini, Calligaris, Cascarino, Boattin; Gunnarsdottir (70' Girelli), Caruso, Grosso; Cantore (70' Echegini), Beerensteyn, Bonansea (71' Garbino)
A disposizione: Aprile, Gama, Salvai, Cafferata, Bellucci,

Thomas
Allenatore: Joseph Adrian Montemurro

FIORENTINA FEMMINILE (4-3-3): Schroffenegger; Erzen, Agard (90' Toniolo), Tortelli, Faerge; Johannsdottir (80' Georgeva), Severini, Catena (90' Cinotti); Janogy (69' Mijatovic), Boquete, Hammarlund (69' Longo)
A disposizione: Baldi, Russo, Spinelli, Lundin
Allenatore: Sebastian De La Fuente
ARBITRO: Mattia Drigo
AMMONITE: 79' Caruso (J); 80' Schroffenegger (F)
ESPULSE: nessuna

27/01/2024 ore 14:30

ROMA FEMMINILE - SAMPDORIA FEMMINILE 2-0
Reti: 15' Linari (R), 67' Greggi (R)
ROMA FEMMINILE (4-3-3): Korpela; Minami, Kumagai, Linari, Sonstevold; Giugliano (90+1' Kramzar), Greggi, Feiersinger (76' Ciccotti); Glionna (90+1' Cimo), Giacinti (54' Viens), Haavi (76' Pilgrim)
A disposizione: Ceasar, Di Guglielmo, Valdezate Testa
Allenatore: Alessandro Spugna
SAMPDORIA FEMMINILE (4-4-2): Tampieri; De Rita, Pisani, Giordano (68' Nagy), Oliviero; Heroum, Benoit, Schatzer, Cuschieri (58' Baldi); Tarenzi (68' Della Peruta V.), Tatiely
A disposizione: Karresmaa, Marenco, Della Peruta T., Brustia, Battelani, Fallico
Allenatore: Salvatore Mango
ARBITRO: Cristiano Ursini
AMMONITE: 61' Giugliano (R); 75' Nagy (S)
ESPULSE: nessuno

28/01/2024 ore 12:30

POMIGLIANO FEMMINILE - MILAN FEMMINILE 0-0
POMIGLIANO FEMMINILE (4-3-2-1): Gavillet; Battistini, Apicella, Caiazzo, Fusini (90' Domi); Di Giammarino, Ferrario, Rabot; Ippolito, Harvey Lynn (74' Novellino); Nambi (61' Arcangeli)
A disposizione: Buhigas, Vingiani, Schettino, Szymanowski, Manca, Babic
Allenatore: Alessandro Caruso

MILAN FEMMINILE (4-3-3): Babb; Bergamaschi (46' Guagni), Mesjasz, Swaby, Soffia; Grimshaw (84' Vigilucci), Mascarello (84' Cernoia), Dubcová; Laurent, Stašková (65' Nadim), Rubio Avila (46' Dompig)
A disposizione: Giuliani, Fusetti, Arrigoni, Marinelli
Allenatore: Davide Corti
ARBITRO: Domenico Leone
AMMONITE: 32' Bergamaschi (M); 82' Ippolito (P)
ESPULSE: nessuna

28/01/2024 ore 15:00

COMO WOMEN - SASSUOLO FEMMINILE 0-1
Reti: 84' Clelland (S)
COMO WOMEN (4-2-3-1): Korenciova; Lundorf Skovsen (59' Zanoli), Rizzon, Lipman, Cecotti; Karlernas, Vaitukaityt? (79' Hilaj); Monnecchi (59' Sevenius), Skorvankova, Martinovic (73' Bergersen Schaathun)
A disposizione: Gilardi, Pastrenge, Bianchi, Picchi
Allenatore: Marco Bruzzano
SASSUOLO FEMMINILE (4-3-3): Durand; Mella, Filangeri, Pleidrup, Philtjens; Pondini (68' Mihelic), Missipo, Prugna; Beccari (11' Sciabica), Kullashi (68' Clelland), Sabatino (90' Monterubbiano)
A disposizione: Lonni, Kresche, Santoro, Brignoli, Tudisco
Allenatore: Gianpiero Piovani
ARBITRO: Edoardo Manedo Mazzoni
AMMONITE: 70' Zanoli (C); 72' Sciabica (S)
ESPULSE: nessuna

27/01/2024 ore 12:30

NAPOLI FEMMINILE - INTER WOMEN 2-3
Reti: 7' Corelli (N), 47' Magull (I), 51' Magull (I), 84' Polli (I), 90+3' Kobayashi (N)
NAPOLI FEMMINILE (4-3-1-2): Bacic; Bertucci (64' Lazaro Torres Del Molino), Di Marino, Pettenuzzo, Pellinghelli; Giai (80' Mauri), Gallazzi, Kobayashi; Chmielinski; Corelli (75' Banusic Meredinho), Del Estal
A disposizione: Beretta, Fabiano, Veritti, Giacobbo, Kajzba
Allenatore: Biagio Seno
INTER WOMEN (3-5-2): Cetinja; Bowen, Alborghetti, Tomter (46' Polli); Merlo, Magull, Junge Pedersen, Santi (25' Csiszár), Robustellini; Cambiaghi (68' Bugeja), Bonfantini (85' Pandini)
A disposizione: Piazza, Capecchi, Fordos, Thogersen, Jelcic
Allenatore: Rita Guarino
ARBITRO: Gabriele Sacchi
AMMONITE: nessuna
ESPULSE: nessuna

15

Sampdoria Femminile	1
Pomigliano Femminile	0
Roma Femminile	3
Juventus Women	1
Sassuolo Femminile	2
Napoli Femminile	0
Milan Femminile	2
Fiorentina Femminile	2
Inter Women	2
Como Women	3

04/02/2024 ore 12:30

SAMPDORIA FEMMINILE-POMIGLIANO FEMMINILE 1-0

Reti: 30' Tatiely (S)

SAMPDORIA FEMMINILE (4-4-2): Tampieri; De Rita, Re, Pisani (90+2' Heroum), Oliviero; Giordano (90+2' Brustia), Benoit, Schatzer, Baldi (73' Cuschieri); Battelani (73' Fallico), Tatiely

A disposizione: Karresmaa, Panzeri, Tarenzi, Nagy, Della Peruta V.

Allenatore: Salvatore Mango

POMIGLIANO FEMMINILE (4-3-2-1): Gavillet; Battistini (89' Manca), Apicella, Rabot, Fusini (72' Novellino); Harvey Lynn (55' Szymanowski), Ferrario, Di Giammarino (89' Domi); Arcangeli (72' Babic), Ippolito; Nambi

A disposizione: Vingiani, Schettino, Buhigas

Allenatore: Alessandro Caruso

ARBITRO: Enrico Gigliotti

AMMONITE: 27' Apicella (P); 43' Harvey Lynn (P); 60' Fusini (P); 61' Tatiely (S); 78' Battistini (P); 90+5' Cuschieri (S)

ESPULSE: nessuno

04/02/2024 ore 16:00

ROMA FEMMINILE - JUVENTUS WOMEN 3-1

Reti: 21' Giugliano (Rig.) (R), 63' Viens (R), 69' Linari (R), 90+2' Thomas (J)

ROMA FEMMINILE (4-1-4-1): Ceasar; Di Guglielmo (87' Bartoli), Minami, Linari, Sonstevold; Kumagai; Glionna (73' Pilgrim), Giugliano, Greggi (85' Troelsgaard), Haavi; Viens (85' Giacinti)

A disposizione: Korpela, Ciccotti, Tomaselli, Feiersinger, Kramzar

Allenatore: Alessandro Spugna

JUVENTUS WOMEN (4-2-3-1): Peyraud-Magnin; Lenzini (79' Gama), Calligaris, Cascarino, Boattin; Caruso, Grosso; Cantore (60' Bonansea), Gunnarsdottir (70' Girelli), Echegini (79' Thomas); Beerensteyn (70' Garbino)

A disposizione: Aprile, Salvai, Palis, Bragonzi

Allenatore: Joseph Adrian Montemurro

ARBITRO: Marco Emmanuele

AMMONITE: 78' Minami (R); 80' Kumagai (R)

ESPULSE: nessuna

03/02/2024 ore 12:30

SASSUOLO FEMMINILE - NAPOLI FEMMINILE 2-0

Reti: 62' Di Bari (Aut.) (N), 79' Pleidrup (S)

SASSUOLO FEMMINILE (4-3-3): Durand; Mella, Filangeri, Pleidrup, Philtjens; Pondini (46' Mihelic), Missipo, Prugna (90+1' Santoro); Clelland (88' Sciabica), Kullashi (90+1' Simon), Sabatino (74' Monterubbiano)

A disposizione: Lonni, Kresche, Passeri, Tudisco

Allenatore: Gianpiero Piovani

NAPOLI FEMMINILE (4-3-3): Bacic; Pellinghelli (76' Bertucci), Di Marino, Di Bari, Kobayashi; Giacobbo (66' Kajzba), Gallazzi, Giai (77' Gianfico); Del Estal (57' Chmielinski), Banusic Meredinho, Corelli (57' Lazaro Torres Del Molino)

A disposizione: Beretta, Veritti, Pettenuzzo, Mauri

Allenatore: Biagio Seno

ARBITRO: Antonio Di Reda

AMMONITE: 78' Di Marino (N); 88' Prugna (S)

ESPULSE: nessuna

03/02/2024 ore 15:00

MILAN FEMMINILE - FIORENTINA FEMMINILE 2-2

Reti: 15' Dubcová (M), 21' Janogy (F), 40' Stašková (M), 51' Agard (F)

MILAN FEMMINILE (4-3-3): Giuliani; Guagni (66' Soffia), Swaby, Piga, Bergamaschi; Grimshaw, Mascarello (85' Vigilucci), Dubcová (85' Dompig); Laurent (86' Marinelli), Stašková, Nadim (46' Ijeh)

A disposizione: Copetti, Fusetti, Cernoia, Rubio Avila

Allenatore: Davide Corti

FIORENTINA FEMMINILE (4-3-3): Baldi; Erzen, Tortelli (39' Spinelli; 46' Toniolo), Agard, Faerge; Johannsdottir (73' Mijatovic), Severini, Catena (73' Cinotti); Janogy, Boquete, Hammarlund (58' Longo)

A disposizione: Schroffenegger, Russo, Tucceri Cimini, Santini

Allenatore: Sebastian De La Fuente

ARBITRO: Edoardo Gianquinto

AMMONITE: 76' Severini (F); 83' Bergamaschi (M); 86' Erzen (F); 88' Mijatovic (F)

ESPULSE: nessuna

03/02/2024 ore 18:00

INTER WOMEN - COMO WOMEN 2-3

Reti: 27' Magull (Rig.) (I), 30' Kajan (C), 47' Kajan (C), 49' Cambiaghi (I), 71' Karlernas (C)

INTER WOMEN (4-3-3): Cetinja; Merlo (86' Thogersen), Alborghetti, Bowen, Robustellini; Magull, Junge Pedersen, Csiszár (86' Jelcic); Cambiaghi, Polli (66' Serturini), Bonfantini

A disposizione: Piazza, Fordos, Tomter, Pandini, Fadda, Bugeja

Allenatore: Rita Guarino

COMO WOMEN (4-2-3-1): Gilardi; Lundorf Skovsen (46' Monnecchi), Rizzon, Lipman, Cecotti (38' Bergersen Schaathun); Hilaj (79' Pastrenge), Vaitukaityt? (82' Sevenius); Karlernas, Picchi (46' Zanoli), Skorvankova; Kajan

A disposizione: Korenciova, Bianchi, Colombo, Martinovic

Allenatore: Marco Bruzzano

ARBITRO: Gioele Iacobellis

AMMONITE: 39' Bonfantini (I); 63' Vaitukaityt? (C); 77' Lipman (C); 90+5' Karlernas (C)

ESPULSE: nessuna

16

Juventus Women	5
Como Women	0
Sassuolo Femminile	1
Milan Femminile	0
Fiorentina Femminile	2
Sampdoria Femminile	1
Napoli Femminile	0
Roma Femminile	1
Pomigliano Femminile	2
Inter Women	6

Tabellini

11/02/2024 ore 18:00

JUVENTUS WOMEN - COMO WOMEN 5-0

Reti: 16' Garbino (J), 33' Girelli (J), 50' Girelli (J), 56' Boattin (J), 85' Thomas (J)

JUVENTUS WOMEN (4-3-3): Peyraud-Magnin; Lenzini (63' Gama), Salvai, Cascarino, Boattin; Caruso (55' Palis), Grosso (63' Thomas), Garbino; Cantore, Girelli (75' Bragonzi), Echegini (75' Pelgander)

A disposizione: Aprile, Calligaris, Bonansea, Beerensteyn

Allenatore: Joseph Adrian Montemurro

COMO WOMEN (4-4-2): Korenciova; Bergersen Schaathun, Rizzon, Lipman, Zanoli (54' Lundorf Skovsen); Monnecchi, Hilaj (61' Pastrenge), Vaitukaityt?, Karlernas (65' Picchi); Kajan (60' Martinovic), Skorvankova (60' Sevenius)

A disposizione: Gilardi, Liva, Bianchi, Colombo

Allenatore: Marco Bruzzano

ARBITRO: Gianluca Catanzaro

AMMONITE: 69' Vaitukaityt? (C)

ESPULSE: nessuna

10/02/2024 ore 18:00

SASSUOLO FEMMINILE - MILAN FEMMINILE 1-0

Reti: 33' Sabatino (Rig.) (S)

SASSUOLO FEMMINILE (4-3-1-2): Durand; Mella, Filangeri, Pleidrup, Philtjens; Pondini, Missipo, Prugna; Kullashi; Clelland (77' Mihelic), Sabatino (62' Beccari; 85' Monterubbiano)

A disposizione: Lonni, Passeri, Santoro, Orsi, Simon, Sciabica

Allenatore: Gianpiero Piovani

MILAN FEMMINILE (4-3-3): Giuliani; Soffia (77' Fusetti), Mesjasz, Piga, Bergamaschi (69' Guagni); Grimshaw, Mascarello (69' Ijeh), Dubcová (46' Laurent); Dompig, Stašková, Nadim (46' Vigilucci)

A disposizione: Babb, Cesarini, Arrigoni, Marinelli

Allenatore: Davide Corti

ARBITRO: Eugenio Scarpa

AMMONITE: 7' Pleidrup (S); 30' Piga (M); 33' Soffia (M); 38' Mesjasz (M)

ESPULSE: a fine partita Laurent (M)

11/02/2024 ore 15:15

FIORENTINA WOMEN'S - SAMPDORIA FEMMINILE 2-1

Reti: 20' Re (Aut.) (S), 80' Johannsdottir (F), 88' Della Peruta V. (S)

FIORENTINA FEMMINILE (4-3-3): Baldi; Erzen, Faerge, Agard, Toniolo; Severini, Cinotti (76' Parisi), Catena (83' Tucceri Cimini); Longo (76' Bellucci), Hammarlund (62' Janogy), Mijatovic (62' Johannsdottir)

A disposizione: Schroffenegger, Russo, Santini Boquete

Allenatore: Sebastian De La Fuente

SAMPDORIA FEMMINILE (4-4-2): Tampieri; Brustia, De Rita, Re, Oliviero; Giordano (81' Tarenzi), Schatzer, Benoit (89' Micheli), Cuschieri (63' Batte-lani); Tatiely, Baldi (81' Della Peruta V.)

A disposizione: Karresmaa, Marenco, Nagy, Della Peruta T., Fallico

Allenatore: Salvatore Mango

ARBITRO: Filippo Colaninno

AMMONITE: 66' Toniolo (F); 83' Severini (F); 84' Baldi (F)

ESPULSE: nessuno

10/02/2024 ore 15:00

NAPOLI FEMMINILE - ROMA FEMMINILE 0-1

Reti: 44' Giugliano (R)

NAPOLI FEMMINILE (4-4-2): Bacic; Pellinghelli, Di Marino, Pettenuzzo, Kobayashi; Bertucci (72' Giacobbo), Giai (66' Mauri), Gallazzi, Chmielinski; Lazaro Torres Del Molino (81' Gianfico), Del Estal (66' Corelli)

A disposizione: Beretta, Fabiano, Di Bari, Veritti, Kajzba

Allenatore: Biagio Seno

ROMA FEMMINILE (4-3-3): Ceasar; Bartoli, Valdezate (78' Troelsgaard), Linari, Di Guglielmo; Kramzar (65' Greggi), Kumagai, Giugliano; Viens, Giacinti (87' Sonstevold), Haavi (78' Pilgrim)

A disposizione: Korpela, Ciccotti, Tomaselli, Feiersinger, Glionna

Allenatore: Alessandro Spugna

ARBITRO: Francesco Zago

AMMONITE: 2' Ceasar (R); 53' Giai (N); 77' Lazaro Torres Del Molino (N); 84' Giacinti (R)

ESPULSE: nessuna

11/02/2024 ore 12:00

POMIGLIANO FEMMINILE - INTER WOMEN 2-6

Reti: 3' Serturini (I), 11' Bugeja (I), 38' Magull (I), 57' Fordos (Aut.) (I), 60' Magull (I), 61' Robustellini (Aut.) (I), 64' Robustellini (I), 76' Jelcic (I)

POMIGLIANO FEMMINILE (4-3-2-1): Gavillet; Battistini, Apicella, Rabot, Fusini; Harvey Lynn, Ferrario (82' Szymanowski), Di Giammarino (69' Domi); Arcangeli (75' Babic),

Ippolito (82' Manca); Novellino (46' Nambi)
A disposizione: Buhigas, Caiazzo, Vingiani, Schettino
Allenatore: Alessandro Caruso
INTER WOMEN (4-3-3): Cetinja; Alborghetti (46' Fordos), Thogersen, Tomter, Robustellini; Magull (64' Pandini), Csiszár (70' Simonetti), Milinkovic; Serturini (80' Bonetti), Polli (64' Jelcic), Bugeja
A disposizione: Piazza, Merlo, Bonfantini, Cambiaghi
Allenatore: Rita Guarino
ARBITRO: Mario Perri
AMMONITE: nessuna
ESPULSE: nessuna

17

GIORNATA

Como Women	0
Fiorentina Femminile	1
Inter Women	0
Juventus Women	2
Napoli Femminile	2
Pomigliano Femminile	0
Roma Femminile	3
Sassuolo Femminile	0
Sampdoria Femminile	1
Milan Femminile	3

Tabellini

14/02/2024 ore 15:00
COMO WOMEN - FIORENTINA FEMMINILE 0-1
Reti: 72' Boquete (F)
COMO WOMEN (4-4-2): Gilardi; Bergersen Schaathun, Rizzon, Lipman, Lundorf Skovsen; Monnecchi, Skorvankova (59' Picchi), Karlernas

(67' Vaitukaityt?), Pastrenge (67' Hilaj); Kajan, Sevenius (76' Martinovic)
A disposizione: Korenciova, Zanoli, Liva, Bianchi, Colombo
Allenatore: Marco Bruzzano
FIORENTINA FEMMINILE (4-3-3): Schroffenegger; Erzen, Faerge, Georgeva (73' Mijatovic), Toniolo; Johannsdottir (65' Parisi), Severini, Catena (74' Bellucci); Longo (79' Tucceri Cimini), Janogy (65' Hammarlund), Boquete
A disposizione: Baldi, Russo, Agard, Cinotti
Allenatore: Sebastian De La Fuente
ARBITRO: Alfredo Iannello
AMMONITE: 30' Lipman (C); 43' Severini (F); 47' Pastrenge (C); 68' Toniolo (F); 90+1' Erzen (F)
ESPULSE: nessuna

14/02/2024 ore 19:00
INTER WOMEN - JUVENTUS WOMEN 0-2
Reti: 7' Echegini (J), 14' Echegini (J)
INTER WOMEN (4-3-3): Cetinja; Thogersen, Alborghetti, Tomter, Robustellini; Magull, Csiszár (75' Polli), Milinkovic; Bonfantini (68' Bugeja), Cambiaghi, Serturini (87' Jelcic)
A disposizione: Piazza, Fordos, Pandini, Simonetti, Bonetti, D'Elia
Allenatore: Rita Guarino
JUVENTUS WOMEN (4-3-3): Peyraud-Magnin; Lenzini (79' Gama), Calligaris, Salvai, Boattin; Echegini (79' Thomas), Grosso (84' Palis), Caruso; Cantore (71' Bonansea), Girelli, Garbino (71' Beerensteyn)
A disposizione: Aprile, Cascarino, Pelgander, Bragonzi
Allenatore: Joseph Adrian Montemurro
ARBITRO: Maria Marotta
AMMONITE: 12' Caruso (J); 27' Magull (I); 57' Boattin (J); 85' Milinkovic (I); 90' Peyraud-Magnin (J)
ESPULSE: nessuna

15/02/2024 ore 20:30
NAPOLI FEMMINILE - POMIGLIANO FEMMINILE 2-0
Reti: 28' Del Estal (N), 32' Di Marino (N)
NAPOLI FEMMINILE (4-4-2): Bacic; Pellinghelli, Pettenuzzo, Di Marino, Kobayashi; Bertucci (62' Giacobbo), Giai, Gallazzi, Chmielinski (90+1' Di Bari); Lazaro Torres Del Molino (90+1' Mauri), Del Estal (83' Corelli)
A disposizione: Beretta, Veritti, Kajzba, Banusic Meredinho, Gianfico
Allenatore: Biagio Seno
POMIGLIANO FEMMINILE (4-3-1-2): Buhigas; Battistini (70' Novellino), Apicella, Caiazzo, Fusini; Rabot (62' Babic), Ferrario, Di Giammarino (87' Harvey Lynn); Ippolito; Nambi (46' Szymanowski), Arcangeli
A disposizione: Gavillet, Vingiani, Schettino, Domi, Manca
Allenatore: Roberto Carannante
ARBITRO: Giuseppe Mucera
AMMONITE: 7' Di Marino (N); 47' Arcangeli (P); 64' Apicella (P); 73' Lazaro Torres Del Molino (N)
ESPULSE: nessuna

13/02/2024 ore 17:00
ROMA FEMMINILE - SASSUOLO FEMMINILE 3-0
Reti: 8' Giacinti (Rig.) (R), 11' Giacinti (R), 51' Giacinti (R)
ROMA FEMMINILE (4-3-3): Ceasar; Bartoli, Linari, Minami, Sonstevold; Giugliano (46' Feiersinger), Kumagai (60' Troelsgaard), Greggi (75' Tomaselli); Viens, Giacinti (61' Pilgrim), Haavi (60' Glionna)
A disposizione: Korpela, Di Guglielmo, Ciccotti, Kramzar
Allenatore: Alessandro Spugna
SASSUOLO FEMMINILE (4-3-1-2): Lonni; Mella, Passeri, Pleidrup, Philtjens; Pondini (67' Prugna), Missipo, Santoro (69' Simon); Kullashi (55' Mihelic); Monterubbiano (55' Sciabica), Sabatino (55' Clelland)

A disposizione: Durand, Kresche, Tudisco, Filangeri
Allenatore: Gianpiero Piovani
ARBITRO: Daniele Virgilio
AMMONITE: nessuna
ESPULSE: nessuna

14/02/2024 ore 15:00
SAMPDORIA FEMMINILE-MILAN FEMMINILE 1-3
Reti: 9' Tarenzi (S), 31' Dompig (M), 53' Rubio Avila (M), 56' Dompig (M)
SAMPDORIA FEMMINILE (4-1-4-1): Tampieri; Heroum, De Rita, Re Oliviero; Benoit; Giordano (73' Della Peruta T.), Schatzer (90' Fallico), Battelani (46' Baldi), Tatiely; Tarenzi (57' Della Peruta V.)
A disposizione: Karresmaa, Marenco, Nagy, Cuschieri, Brustia
Allenatore: Salvatore Mango
MILAN FEMMINILE (4-3-3): Giuliani; Guagni, Piga (46' Fusetti), Mesjasz, Soffia; Dubcova, Rubio Avila (71' Mascarello), Grimshaw; Dompig (82' Vigilucci), Nadim (71' Ijeh), Marinelli (71' Staskova)
A disposizione: Babb, Bergamaschi, Cesarini, Arrigoni
Allenatore: Davide Corti
ARBITRO: Simone Gauzolino
AMMONITE: 6' Re (S); 83' Mesjasz (M)
ESPULSE: nessuno

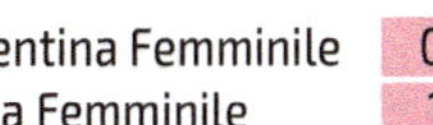

18

GIORNATA

| Milan Femminile | 2 |
| Inter Women | 1 |

| Fiorentina Femminile | 0 |
| Roma Femminile | 1 |

| Juventus Women | 4 |
| Napoli Femminile | 1 |

| Pomigliano Femminile | 3 |
| Como Women | 4 |

| Sassuolo Femminile | 2 |
| Sampdoria Femminile | 0 |

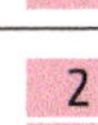
Tabellini

18/02/2024 ore 17:00
MILAN FEMMINILE - INTER WOMEN 2-1
Reti: 9' Alborghetti (Aut.) (I), 34' Stašková (M), 45' Serturini (I)
MILAN FEMMINILE (4-3-3): Giuliani; Guagni, Piga, Mesjasz, Bergamaschi; Grimshaw (64' Vigilucci), Mascarello, Dubcová; Dompig (82' Rubio Avila), Stašková (67' Soffia), Marinelli (83' Ijeh)
A disposizione: Babb, Fusetti, Cernoia, Asllani, Arrigoni
Allenatore: Davide Corti
INTER WOMEN (4-3-3): Cetinja; Thogersen (78' Bonfantini), Alborghetti, Tomter (78' Bonetti), Robustellini (16' Fordos); Magull, Csiszár (90' Simonetti), Milinkovic; Bugeja (46' Polli), Cambiaghi, Serturini
A disposizione: Piazza, Capecchi, Pandini, Jelcic
Allenatore: Rita Guarino
ARBITRO: Matteo Centi
AMMONITE: 61' Milinkovic (I)
ESPULSE: nessuna

17/02/2024 ore 15:00
FIORENTINA FEMMINILE - ROMA FEMMINILE 0-1
Reti: 43' Giugliano (R)
FIORENTINA FEMMINILE (4-3-3): Schroffenegger; Erzen (75' Toniolo), Georgeva, Agard, Faerge; Parisi (59' Johannsdottir), Cinotti (75' Bellucci), Catena; Boquete, Hammarlund (59' Janogy), Longo (82' Mijatovic)
A disposizione: Baldi, Russo, Zaghini, Tucceri Cimini
Allenatore: Sebastian De La Fuente
ROMA FEMMINILE (4-3-3):

Ceasar; Di Guglielmo, Minami, Linari, Sonstevold; Giugliano (73' Troelsgaard), Kumagai, Greggi; Viens (90+2' Glionna), Giacinti (64' Pilgrim), Haavi
A disposizione: Korpela, Valdezate, Bartoli, Ciccotti, Tomaselli, Kramzar
Allenatore: Alessandro Spugna
ARBITRO: Giorgio Vergaro
AMMONITE: nessuna
ESPULSE: nessuna

18/02/2024 ore 12:30
JUVENTUS WOMEN - NAPOLI FEMMINILE 4-1
Reti: 9' Girelli (Rig.) (J), 17' Thomas (J), 45' Grosso (J), 90+1' Thomas (J), 90+4' Banusic Meredinho (Rig.) (N)
JUVENTUS WOMEN (4-3-3): Peyraud-Magnin; Lenzini (65' Gama), Calligaris, Salvai (75' Cascarino), Boattin; Caruso (65' Palis), Grosso, Garbino; Beerensteyn (65' Bonansea), Girelli (75' Bragonzi), Thomas
A disposizione: Aprile, Echegini, Nyström, Cantore
Allenatore: Joseph Adrian Montemurro
NAPOLI FEMMINILE (4-4-2): Bacic; Pellinghelli (69' Di Bari), Pettenuzzo, Di Marino (76' Veritti), Kobayashi; Bertucci (56' Banusic Meredinho), Giai (46' Giacobbo), Gallazzi, Chmielinski; Lazaro Torres Del Molino (46' Corelli), Del Estal
A disposizione: Beretta, Mauri, Kajzba, Gianfico
Allenatore: Biagio Seno
ARBITRO: Giorgio Bozzetto
AMMONITE: 90+2' Banusic Meredinho (N)
ESPULSE: nessuna

18/02/2024 ore 15:00
POMIGLIANO FEMMINILE - COMO WOMEN 3-4
Reti: 9' Ippolito (P), 18' Apicella (P), 58' Martinovic (C), 60' Rizzon (C), 63' Kajan (Rig.) (C), 69' Arcangeli (P), 90+5' Martinovic (C)
POMIGLIANO FEMMINILE (3-5-2): Buhigas; Battisti-

Classifica

La Serie A Femminile 2023-24 conferma lo strapotere della **Roma**. La formazione diretta da Alessandro Spugna si aggiudica il campionato vincendo 23 dei 26 impegni sostenuti.

Alle spalle delle giallorosse, vincitrici anche della Coppa Italia, si piazza nuovamente la **Juventus**. A determinare gran parte del distacco finale tra le due squadre è il bilancio dei confronti diretti: tre successi a uno per la compagine capitolina.

Dietro le due corazzate troviamo la **Fiorentina** di Sebastian De La Fuente che si garantisce l'accesso alla prossima Uefa Women's Champions League.

A seguire troviamo **Sassuolo, Inter, Milan, Como e Sampdoria**.

Il **Napoli** si assicura la permanenza nella massima serie prevalendo nello spareggio salvezza contro la Ternana.

Il **Pomigliano**, dopo tre partecipazioni, saluta la Serie A.

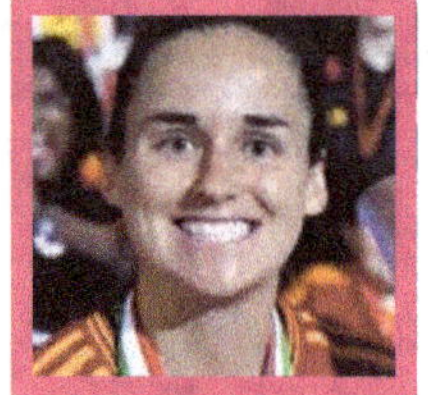

13 Evelyne Viens
Roma Femminile

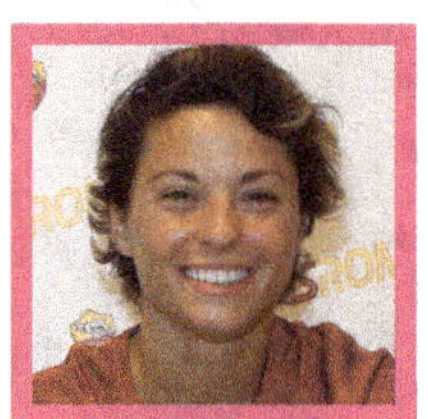

12 Valentina Giacinti
Roma Femminile

Squadra	Pt	G	V	N	P	GF	GS	PtC	GC
Roma Femminile	51	18	17	0	1	51	11	27	9
Juventus Women	43	18	14	1	3	47	16	22	9
Fiorentina Femminile	39	18	12	3	3	36	19	21	9
Sassuolo Femminile	26	18	8	2	8	20	20	10	9
Inter Women	26	18	8	2	8	28	29	14	9
Milan Femminile	21	18	5	6	7	22	22	13	9
Como Women	21	18	6	3	9	20	33	8	9
Sampdoria Femminile	18	18	5	3	10	12	29	7	9
Napoli Femminile	6	18	1	3	14	11	36	4	9
Pomigliano Femminile	6	18	1	3	14	14	46	4	9

LEGENDA STATISTICHE GENERALI: Pt Punti. **G** Partite giocate. **V** Partite vinte. **N** Partite pareggiate. **P** Partite perse. **GF** Gol fatti. **GS** Gol subiti - **STATISTICHE IN CASA: PtC** Punti in casa. **GC** Partite giocate in casa. **VC** Partite vinte in casa. **NC** Partite pareggiate in casa. **PC** Partite perse in casa.

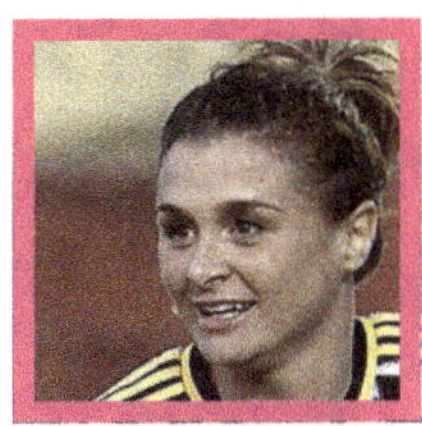

11 **Cristiana Girelli**
Juventus Women

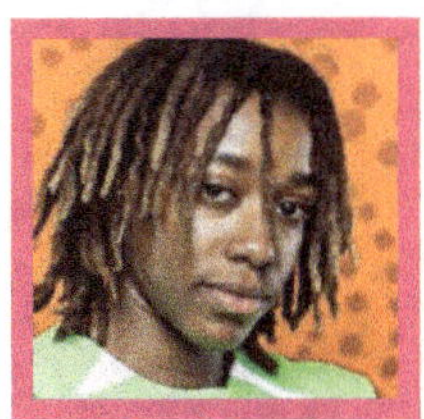

10 **Jennifer Echegini**
Juventus Women *

* A pari merito con Manuela Giugliano (Roma Femminile), ma con miglior rendimento

ni, Apicella, Caiazzo; Harvey Lynn, Ferrario, Di Giammarino, Rabot, Fusini (65' Novellino); Ippolito (90+4' Babic), Arcangeli (90' Nambi)
A disposizione: Gavillet, Vingiani, Schettino, Domi, Szymanowski, Manca
Allenatore: Roberto Carannante
COMO WOMEN (4-2-3-1): Korenciova; Lundorf Skovsen (46' Zanoli), Rizzon, Lipman (88' Hilaj), Bergersen Schaathun; Pastrenge (56' Martinovic), Vaitukaityt? (64' Picchi); Skorvankova, Karlernas (46' Sevenius), Monnecchi; Kajan
A disposizione: Gilardi, Bianchi, Regazzoli, Colombo
Allenatore: Marco Bruzzano
ARBITRO: Valerio Pezzopane
AMMONITE: 20' Rabot (P); 27' Apicella (P); 27' Karlernas (C); 39' Lundorf Skovsen (C); 42' Fusini (P); 77' Skorvankova (C); 90+6' Martinovic (C)
ESPULSE: nessuna

17/02/2024 ore 12:30
SASSUOLO FEMMINILE-SAMPDORIA FEMMINILE 2-0
Reti: 53' Kullashi (Sas), 69' Sabatino (Sas)
SASSUOLO-FEMMINILE (4-3-1-2): Durand; Mella, Filangeri, Pleidrup, Philtjens; Pondini, Missipo (46' Mihelic), Prugna (82' Tudisco); Kullashi; Clelland (67' Passeri), Sabatino (82' Sciabica)
A disposizione: Lonni, Kresche, Santoro, Simon, Monterubbiano
Allenatore: Gianpiero Piovani
SAMPDORIA FEMMINILE (4-5-1): Karresmaa; Brustia, De Rita (46' Marenco), Re, Oliviero; Giordano (68' Battelani), Schatzer, Benoit (67' Fallico), Cuschieri (78' Tarenzi), Tatiely; Della Peruta T. (57' Baldi)
A disposizione: Tampieri, Heroum, Nagy, Della Peruta V.
Allenatore: Salvatore Mango
ARBITRO: Fabio Rosario Luongo
AMMONITE: 29' Tatiely (Sam)
ESPULSE: nessuno

VC	NC	PC	GFC	GSC	PtT	GT	VT	NT	PT	GFT	GST	M.I.	
9	0	0	27	4	24	9	8	0	1	24	7	15	
7	1	1	31	8	21	9	7	0	2	16	8	7	accedono a Poule Scudetto
7	0	2	18	8	18	9	5	3	1	18	11	3	
3	1	5	9	10	16	9	5	1	3	11	10	-10	
4	2	3	11	9	12	9	4	0	5	17	20	-10	
3	4	2	16	14	8	9	2	2	5	6	8	-15	
2	2	5	6	11	13	9	4	1	4	14	22	-15	accedono a Poule Salvezza
2	1	6	4	17	11	9	3	2	4	8	12	-18	
1	1	7	7	15	2	9	0	2	7	4	21	-30	
1	1	7	10	26	2	9	0	2	7	4	20	-30	

GFC Gol fatti in casa. **GSC** Gol subiti in casa. **STATISTICHE IN TRASFERTA: PtT** Punti in trasferta. **GT** Partite giocate in trasferta. **VT** Partite vinte in trasferta. **NT** Partite pareggiate in trasferta. **PT** Partite perse in trasferta. **GFT** Goal fatti in trasferta. **GST** Goal subiti in trasferta. **M.I.** Media inglese

Giornate e Tabellini

1
GIORNATA

Inter Women	3
Juventus Women	3
Sassuolo Femminile	1
Fiorentina Femminile	0

Tabellini

17/03/2024 ore 16:00

INTER WOMEN-JUVENTUS WOMEN 3-3
Reti: 17' Simonetti (I), 38' Girelli (J), 50' Cambiaghi (I), 58' Caruso (J), 63' Echegini (J), 86' Serturini (I)
INTER WOMEN (4-3-3): Durante; Thogersen, Fordos, Bowen, Tomter (72' Robustellini); Milinkovic, Csiszar (78' Jelcic), Simonetti (64' Magull); Bonfantini (64' Bugeja), Cambiaghi (72' Polli), Serturini
A disposizione: Cetinja, Pandini, Fadda
Allenatore: Rita Guarino
JUVENTUS WOMEN (4-3-3): Peyraud-Magnin; Lenzini, Salvai, Calligaris, Cascarino; Grosso, Girelli (74' Gunnarsdottir), Caruso; Bragonzi (59' Echegini), Thomas (82' Bonansea), Beerensteyn (74' Garbino)
A disposizione: Aprile, Gama,

Cafferata, Gallina, Nystrom
Allenatore: Giuseppe Zappella
ARBITRO: Andrea Ancora
AMMONITE: 69' Fordos (I); 90+6' Lenzini (J)
ESPULSE: nessuno

16/03/2024 ore 15:00

SASSUOLO FEMMINILE-FIORENTINA FEMMINILE 1-0
Reti: 90+1' Beccari (S)
SASSUOLO FEMMINILE (4-3-3): Durand; Orsi, Filangeri, Pleidrup, Philtjens; Pondini (80' Simon), Missipo, Prugna; Sabatino (71' Beccari), Kullashi (46' Mihelic), Clelland (88' Monterubbiano)
A disposizione: Kresche, Passeri, Santoro, Jane, Sciabica
Allenatore: Gianpiero Piovani
FIORENTINA FEMMINILE (4-4-2): Baldi; Erzen (62' Tucceri Cimini), Agard, Georgeva, Faerge; Mijatovic (61' Bellucci), Johannsdottir (62' Lundin), Severini, Catena; Janogy (85' Tortelli), Longo (78' Hammarlund)
A disposizione: Schroffenegger, Toniolo, Cinotti, Parisi
Allenatore: Sebastian De La Fuente
ARBITRO: Alberto Poli
AMMONITE: 45' Severini (F)
ESPULSE: nessuno

2
GIORNATA

Fiorentina Femminile	0
Inter Women	3
Roma Femminile	3
Sassuolo Femminile	0

Tabellini

24/03/2024 ore 15:00

FIORENTINA FEMMINILE-INTER WOMEN 0-3
Reti: 8' Serturini (I), 61' Magull (I), 68' Bonfantini (I)
FIORENTINA FEMMINILE (4-3-3): Schroffenegger; Tortelli, Agard (61' Parisi), Georgeva, Faerge; Erzen (70' Toniolo), Johannsdottir (70' Mijatovic), Severini; Janogy (82' Lundin), Boquete, Longo (61' Hammarlund)
A disposizione: Baldi, Tucceri Cimini, Cinotti, Bellucci
Allenatore: Sebastian De La Fuente
INTER WOMEN (4-3-3): Durante (72' Cetinja); Thogersen, Bowen, Fordos, Robustellini (82' Tomter); Milinkovic, Csiszar (66' Simonetti), Magull; Bonfantini, Cambiaghi (66' Polli), Serturini (82' Bugeja)
A disposizione: Alborghetti,

Pandini, Bonetti, Jelcic
Allenatore: Rita Guarino
ARBITRO: Andrea Calzavara
AMMONITE: 63' Tortelli (F);
68' Robustellini (I); 69' Schroffenegger (F); 74' Milinkovic (I)
ESPULSE: nessuno

23/03/2024 ore 15:00
ROMA FEMMINILE-SASSUOLO FEMMINILE 3-0
Reti: 33' Giugliano (R), 50' Giugliano (Rig.) (R), 58' Giacinti (R)
ROMA FEMMINILE (4-3-3):
Ceasar; Bartoli, Linari, Minami, Sonstevold; Giugliano (73' Feiersinger), Kumagai (73' Troelsgaard), Greggi (82' Tomaselli); Viens (61' Pilgrim), Giacinti, Haavi (61' Di Guglielmo)
A disposizione: Korpela, Valdezate, Ciccotti, Cimo
Allenatore: Alessandro Spugna
SASSUOLO FEMMINILE
(4-3-1-2): Durand; Orsi, Filangeri (68' Simon), Pleidrup, Philtjens; Pondini, Missipo (74' Jane), Prugna (68' Mihelic); Kullashi; Clelland (56' Sabatino), Beccari (46' Sciabica)
A disposizione: Lonni, Passeri, Santoro, Monterubbiano
Allenatore: Gianpiero Piovani
ARBITRO: Maria Marotta
AMMONITE: 30' Pleidrup (S); 45+1' Missipo (S); 71' Linari (R)
ESPULSE: nessuno

3

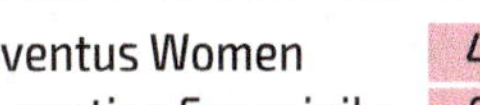

Inter Women	1
Roma Femminile	2

Juventus Women	4
Fiorentina Femminile	0

Tabellini

29/03/2024 ore 18:30
INTER WOMEN - ROMA FEMMINILE 1-2
Reti: 6' Kumagai (R), 60' Bonfantini (I), 89' Troelsgaard (R)
INTER WOMEN (4-3-3):
Cetinja; Robustellini, Fordos, Bowen, Thogersen ; Magull, Csiszar (82' Junge Pedersen), Milinkovic (61' Simonetti); Serturini, Cambiaghi, Bonfantini (75' Bugeja)
A disposizione: Piazza, Alborghetti, Trevisan, Tomter, Pandini
Allenatore: Rita Guarino
ROMA FEMMINILE (4-3-3):
Ceasar; Bartoli, Linari, Minami, Di Guglielmo (65' Sonstevold); Greggi (76' Troelsgaard), Kumagai, Giugliano; Haavi, Giacinti (90+3' Feiersinger), Viens (65' Pilgrim)
A disposizione: Korpela, Valdezate, Ciccotti, Tomaselli, Cimo
Allenatore: Alessandro Spugna
ARBITRO: Andrea Zanotti
AMMONITE: 72' Minami (R)
ESPULSE: nessuno

30/03/2024 ore 15:00
JUVENTUS WOMEN-FIORENTINA FEMMINILE 4-0
Reti: 10' Grosso (J), 13' Echegini (J), 55' Echegini (J), 61' Echegini (J)
JUVENTUS WOMEN (4-3-3):
Peyraud-Magnin; Gama, Lenzini, Calligaris, Boattin; Caruso (63' Gunnarsdottir), Grosso, Echegini (75' Garbino); Girelli (83' Nystrom), Thomas (63' Cantore; 75' Bonansea), Beerensteyn
A disposizione: Aprile, Cascarino, Salvai, Bragonzi
Allenatore: Giuseppe Zappella
FIORENTINA FEMMINILE
(4-4-2): Baldi; Erzen (76' Toniolo), Georgeva, Tortelli, Faerge; Janogy, Johannsdottir (63' Mijatovic), Severini (84' Cinotti), Longo (76' Lundin); Hammarlund (63' Bellucci), Boquete

A disposizione: Schroffenegger, Tucceri Cimini, Agard, Parisi
Allenatore: Sebastian De La Fuente
ARBITRO: Carlo Rinaldi
AMMONITE: 69' Longo (F); 88' Bonansea (J)
ESPULSE: nessuno

4

GIORNATA

Roma Femminile	2
Juventus Women	1

Sassuolo Femminile	2
Inter Women	1

Tabellini

15/04/2024 ore 18:00
ROMA FEMMINILE-JUVENTUS WOMEN 2-1
Reti: 5' Pilgrim (R), 47' Girelli (J), 85' Viens (R)
ROMA FEMMINILE (4-3-3):
Ceasar; Bartoli, Minami, Linari, Sonstevold; Giugliano (90+3' Valdezate), Kumagai, Greggi (83' Troelsgaard); Pilgrim (83' Feiersinger), Giacinti (60' Viens), Haavi
A disposizione: Merolla, Ohrstrom, Testa, Ciccotti, Tomaselli
Allenatore: Alessandro Spugna
JUVENTUS WOMEN (4-3-3):
Peyraud-Magnin; Boattin, Calligaris, Salvai, Lenzini (75' Gama); Echegini (84' Cascarino), Caruso (59' Gunnarsdottir), Grosso; Beerensteyn, Thomas (59' Bonansea), Girelli (75' Cantore)
A disposizione: Aprile, Cafferata, Palis, Nystrom
Allenatore: Giuseppe Zappella

ARBITRO: Lorenzo Maccarini
AMMONITE: 54' Caruso (J); 72' Bonansea (J); 80' Bonansea (J); 82' Kumagai (R)
ESPULSE: 80' Bonansea (J)

13/04/2024 ore 15:00

SASSUOLO FEMMINILE-INTER WOMEN 2-1

Reti: 47' Magull (Rig.) (I), 50' Sabatino (S), 66' Clelland (S)
SASSUOLO FEMMINILE (4-3-1-2): Durand; Orsi (46' Simon), Filangeri, Pleidrup, Philtjens; Pondini (64' Passeri), Jane (77' Zamanian Le Loc'h Bakhtiari), Prugna; Kullashi (58' Missipo); Clelland, Sabatino (64' Beccari)
A disposizione: Lonni, Mihelic, Iriguchi, Monterubbiano
Allenatore: Gianpiero Piovani
INTER WOMEN (4-3-3): Cetinja; Thogersen, Tomter, Fordos, Robustellini; Milinkovic, Csiszar (70' Junge Pedersen), Magull; Bonfantini (90+3' Bowen), Polli (60' Cambiaghi), Bugeja (70' Bonetti)
A disposizione: Piazza, Battilama, Simonetti, Pavan, D'Elia
Allenatore: Rita Guarino
ARBITRO: Alessandro Silvestri
AMMONITE: 13' Orsi (S); 25' Kullashi (S)
ESPULSE: nessuno

5

GIORNATA

| Fiorentina Femminile | 0 |
| Roma Femminile | 0 |

| Juventus Women | 2 |
| Sassuolo Femminile | 1 |

Tabellini

20/04/2024 ore 16:15

FIORENTINA FEMMINILE-ROMA FEMMINILE 0-0

FIORENTINA FEMMINILE (4-4-2): Schroffenegger; Toniolo (90+1' Tucceri Cimini), Georgeva, Tortelli (80' Breitner), Faerge; Janogy, Catena, Severini, Cinotti (90+2' Parisi); Hammarlund (79' Bellucci), Boquete
A disposizione: Baldi, Russo, Spinelli, Agard, Lundin
Allenatore: Sebastian De La Fuente
ROMA FEMMINILE (4-5-1): Ceasar; Bartoli (72' Valdezate), Minami, Linari, Sonstevold; Haavi, Greggi, Kumagai, Feiersinger (59' Troelsgaard), Pilgrim (66' Giacinti); Viens
A disposizione: Ohrstrom, Giugliano, Ciccotti, Tomaselli, Cimo, Glionna
Allenatore: Alessandro Spugna
ARBITRO: Carlo Rinaldi
AMMONITE: 42' Minami (R)
ESPULSE: nessuno

20/04/2024 ore 14:30

JUVENTUS WOMEN-SASSUOLO FEMMINILE 2-1

Reti: 55' Beccari (S), 68' Boattin (J), 80' Nystrom (J)
JUVENTUS WOMEN (4-3-3): Peyraud-Magnin; Lenzini, Gama (75' Cafferata), Salvai, Boattin; Echegini (62' Thomas), Gunnarsdottir, Grosso (86' Palis); Cantore (62' Nystrom), Girelli (86' Bragonzi), Beerensteyn
A disposizione: Aprile, Cascarino, Calligaris, Nava
Allenatore: Giuseppe Zappella
SASSUOLO FEMMINILE (4-3-3): Durand; Orsi, Filangeri, Pleidrup, Philtjens; Jane, Missipo (84' Monterubbiano), Pondini (84' Mihelic); Zamanian Le Loc'h Bakhtiari (53' Clelland), Sabatino (63' Kullashi), Beccari
A disposizione: Lonni, Passeri, Simon, Prugna, Sciabica
Allenatore: Gianpiero Piovani
ARBITRO: Gianluca Renzi

AMMONITE: 30' Lenzini (J); 67' Beccari (S)
ESPULSE: nessuno

6

GIORNATA

| Juventus Women | 0 |
| Inter Women | 2 |

| Fiorentina Femminile | 4 |
| Sassuolo Femminile | 4 |

Tabellini

26/04/2024 ore 20:30

JUVENTUS WOMEN-INTER WOMEN 0-2

Reti: 19' Polli (I), 44' Bugeja (I)
JUVENTUS WOMEN (4-2-3-1): Peyraud-Magnin; Lenzini, Cafferata (71' Echegini), Calligaris (37' Salvai), Cascarino; Gunnarsdottir, Grosso; Cantore (62' Thomas), Girelli, Bonansea (62' Beerensteyn); Nystrom (46' Caruso)
A disposizione: Aprile, Gama, Boattin, Bragonzi
Allenatore: Giuseppe Zappella
INTER WOMEN (4-3-3): Cetinja; Thogersen, Bowen, Fordos, Robustellini; Milinkovic, Junge Pedersen (70' Csiszar), Magull (78' Simonetti); Bonfantini (85' Pavan), Polli (70' Jelcic), Bugeja (85' Alborghetti)
A disposizione: Piazza, Battilama, Pandini, Bonetti
Allenatore: Rita Guarino
ARBITRO: Gabriele Sacchi
AMMONITE: 53' Robustellini (I); 76' Csiszar (I)
ESPULSE: nessuno

27/04/2024 ore 18:00

FIORENTINA FEMMINILE-SASSUOLO FEMMINILE 4-4

Reti: 18' Janogy (F), 30' Prugna (S), 32' Hammarlund (F), 35' Janogy (F), 43' Severini (F), 77' Sabatino (S), 82' Missipo (S), 90+1' Sciabica (S)

FIORENTINA FEMMINILE (4-2-3-1): Schroffenegger; Toniolo (68' Tucceri Cimini), Georgeva, Agard, Faerge; Cinotti (75' Parisi), Severini; Janogy (81' Breitner), Boquete, Catena; Hammarlund (68' Longo)
A disposizione: Baldi, Spinelli, Bellucci, Johannsdottir, Lundin
Allenatore: Sebastian De La Fuente
SASSUOLO FEMMINILE (4-3-1-2): Durand; Orsi, Filangeri, Pleidrup, Philtjens; Pondini (67' Missipo), Zamanian Le Loc'h Bakhtiari (46' Beccari), Clelland (68' Mihelic); Kullashi (78' Monterubbiano); Sabatino, Prugna (90' Sciabica)
A disposizione: Lonni, Kresche, Santoro, Passeri
Allenatore: Gianpiero Piovani
ARBITRO: Antonio Di Reda
AMMONITE: 3' Toniolo (F); 41' Orsi (S); 45' Cinotti (F); 70' Kullashi (S)
ESPULSE: nessuno

GIORNATA

Inter Women	2
Fiorentina Femminile	2
Sassuolo Femminile	5
Roma Femminile	6

Tabellini

01/05/2024 ore 12:30
INTER WOMEN-FIORENTINA FEMMINILE 2-2
Marcatori: 40' Magull (Rig.) (I), 48' Bonfantini (I), 50' Severini (F), 90+6' Boquete (Rig.) (F)

INTER WOMEN (4-3-3): Cetinja; Bowen, Fordos, Alborghetti, Robustellini; Milinkovic, Csiszar (67' Junge Pedersen), Magull; Bonfantini, Polli (68' Jelcic), Bugeja (86' Tomter)
A disposizione: Piazza, Battilama, Pandini, Simonetti, Pavan, Bonetti
Allenatore: Rita Guarino
FIORENTINA FEMMINILE (4-3-1-2): Baldi; Faerge, Agard, Georgeva, Toniolo (79' Tucceri Cimini); Cinotti (61' Johannsdottir), Severini, Catena; Boquete; Janogy (79' Lundin), Hammarlund (71' Longo)
A disposizione: Russo, Spinelli, Breitner, Parisi, Bellucci
Allenatore: Sebastian De La Fuente
ARBITRO: Stefano Milone
AMMONITE: 28' Toniolo (F); 45+3' Csiszar (I); 73' Bonfantini (I); 74' Severini (F)
ESPULSE: nessuna

01/05/2024 ore 15:00
SASSUOLO FEMMINILE-ROMA FEMMINILE 5-6
Marcatori: 5' Giacinti (R), 11' Giacinti (R), 19' Giugliano (R), 23' Clelland (S), 47' Glionna (R), 60' Sabatino (S), 62' Viens (R), 74' Kullashi (S), 75' Clelland (S), 77' Monterubbiano (S), 80' Feiersinger (R)

SASSUOLO FEMMINILE (4-3-3): Durand; Orsi, Filangeri, Pleidrup, Jane (46' Pondini); Missipo (37' Mihelic), Santoro (66' Passeri), Prugna (63' Kullashi); Clelland, Beccari (66' Monterubbiano), Sabatino
A disposizione: Lonni, Kresche, Simon, Zamanian Le Loc'h Bakhtiari
Allenatore: Gianpiero Piovani
ROMA FEMMINILE (3-4-1-2): Ceasar; Valdezate, Kumagai, Minami; Sonstevold (46' Pellegrino Cimo), Troelsgaard (67' Ciccotti), Giugliano (79' Greggi), Tomaselli (51' Feiersinger); Glionna; Viens, Giacinti (66' Galli)

A disposizione: Ohrstrom, Linari, Haavi, Pilgrim
Allenatore: Alessandro Spugna
ARBITRO: Fabrizio Ramondino
AMMONITE: 26' Troelsgaard (R)
ESPULSE: nessuna

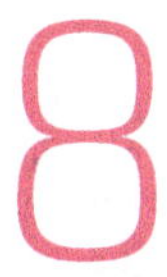

GIORNATA

Roma Femminile	4
Inter Women	3
Fiorentina Femminile	0
Juventus Women	2

Tabellini

05/05/2024 ore 12:30
ROMA FEMMINILE-INTER WOMEN 4-3
Marcatori: 15' Viens (R), 31' Linari (Aut.) (R), 35' Magull (I), 37' Kumagai (R), 44' Bonfantini (I), 75' Viens (R), 80' Giacinti (R)

ROMA FEMMINILE (4-3-3): Ceasar; Sonstevold, Linari, Valdezate (69' Di Guglielmo), Minami; Giugliano (85' Tomaselli), Kumagai (57' Troelsgaard), Greggi (69' Feiersinger); Haavi, Viens, Pilgrim (46' Giacinti)
A disposizione: Merolla, Ohrstrom, Glionna, Pellegrino Cimo
Allenatore: Alessandro Spugna
INTER WOMEN (4-3-3): Cetinja; Bowen, Alborghetti (65' Tomter), Thogersen, Robustellini (72' Simonetti); Milinkovic, Csiszar (90' Junge Pedersen), Magull (90' Bonetti); Bonfantini, Polli, Bugeja (73' Pandini)
A disposizione: Piazza, Pa-

van, Tironi, Jelcic
Allenatore: Rita Guarino
ARBITRO: Giuseppe Maria Manzo
AMMONITE: 48' Minami (R); 76' Polli (I)
ESPULSE: nessuna

06/05/2024 ore 18:00
FIORENTINA FEMMINILE-JUVENTUS WOMEN 0-2
Marcatori: 43' Cantore (J), 87' Bonansea (J)
FIORENTINA FEMMINILE (4-2-3-1): Baldi; Faerge, Georgeva (87' Agard), Spinelli, Tucceri Cimini; Parisi (65' Severini), Johannsdottir (77' Boquete); Bellucci, Lundin (64' Hammarlund), Catena (77' Cinotti); Longo
A disposizione: Bartalini, Russo, Janogy, Santini
Allenatore: Sebastian De La Fuente
JUVENTUS WOMEN (4-3-3): Aprile; Cascarino, Gama (77' Lenzini), Salvai, Boattin; Echegini (84' Pelgander), Gunnarsdottir, Caruso; Cantore (84' Bragonzi), Girelli (65' Beerensteyn), Thomas (76' Bonansea)
A disposizione: Peyraud-Magnin, Cafferata, Palis, Grosso
Allenatore: Paolo Beruatto
ARBITRO: Jules Roland Andeng Tona Mbei
AMMONITE: 35' Longo (F); 53' Catena (F); 80' Gunnarsdottir (J)
ESPULSE: nessuna

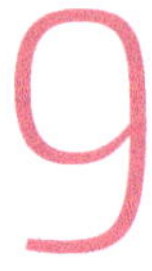

9
GIORNATA

Juventus Women	3
Roma Femminile	1
Inter Women	2
Sassuolo Femminile	4

Tabellini

13/05/2024 ore 18:00
JUVENTUS WOMEN-ROMA FEMMINILE 3-1
Marcatori: 6' Cantore (J), 49' Viens (R), 62' Cantore (J), 90+6' Echegini (J)
JUVENTUS WOMEN (4-4-2): Aprile; Lenzini, Calligaris, Cascarino, Boattin; Bonansea (77' Thomas), Gunnarsdottir, Grosso (63' Beerensteyn), Caruso; Cantore (78' Bragonzi), Girelli (63' Echegini)
A disposizione: Peyraud-Magnin, Gama, Cafferata, Palis, Pelgander
Allenatore: Paolo Beruatto
ROMA FEMMINILE (4-3-3): Ceasar; Di Guglielmo (72' Bartoli), Minami, Linari, Sonstevold; Greggi (57' Troelsgaard), Kumagai (57' Giugliano), Feiersinger; Viens, Giacinti (73' Tomaselli), Glionna (40' Haavi)
A disposizione: Korpela, Valdezate, Ciccotti, Pellegrino Cimo
Allenatore: Alessandro Spugna
ARBITRO: Cristiano Ursini
AMMONITE: 82' Viens (R); 90+4' Thomas (J)
ESPULSE: nessuna

12/05/2024 ore 15:00
INTER WOMEN-SASSUOLO FEMMINILE 2-4
Marcatori: 5' Prugna (S), 20' Clelland (S), 45+7' Clelland (Rig.) (S), 55' Clelland (S), 66' Bugeja (I), 68' Polli (I)
INTER WOMEN (4-3-3): Cetinja; Thogersen, Bowen, Alborghetti, Robustellini; Milinkovic (35' Csiszar), Junge Pedersen (36' Simonetti), Magull; Bonfantini (79' Bonetti), Polli (78' Jelcic), Bugeja (78' Pandini)

Classifica

Squadra	Pt	G	V	N	P	GF	GS	PtC	GC
Roma Femminile	70	26	23	1	2	74	24	39	13
Juventus Women	59	26	19	2	5	65	27	31	13
Fiorentina Femminile	42	26	12	6	8	42	40	23	13
Sassuolo Femminile	36	26	11	3	12	39	41	16	13
Inter Women	34	26	10	4	12	45	46	16	13

LEGENDA STATISTICHE GENERALI: Pt Punti. **G** Partite giocate. **V** Partite vinte. **N** Partite pareggiate. **P** Partite perse. **GF** Gol fatti. **GS** Gol subiti - **STATISTICHE IN CASA: PtC** Punti in casa. **GC** Partite giocate in casa. **VC** Partite vinte in casa. **NC** Partite pareggiate in casa. **PC** Partite perse in casa.

A disposizione: Piazza, Merlo, Tomter, Pavan
Allenatore: Rita Guarino
SASSUOLO FEMMINILE (4-3-3): Durand; Orsi, Filangeri, Pleidrup, Philtjens; Pondini (90' Simon), Passeri (70' Zamanian Le Loc'h Bakhtiari), Prugna; Beccari (70' Santoro), Kullashi (59' Monterubbiano), Clelland (59' Sabatino)
A disposizione: Lonni, Kresche, Mihelic, Jane
Allenatore: Gianpiero Piovani
ARBITRO: Francesco D'Eusanio
AMMONITE: 41' Simonetti (I); 49' Passeri (S); 88' Orsi (S); 90+4' Csiszar (I)
ESPULSE: nessuna

10

Roma Femminile	5
Fiorentina Femminile	0
Sassuolo Femminile	2
Juventus Women	3

19/05/2024 ore 14:30
ROMA FEMMINILE-FIORENTINA FEMMINILE 5-0
Marcatori: 36' Minami (R), 52' Troelsgaard (R), 58' Giacinti (R), 80' Giacinti (R), 84' Viens (R)
ROMA FEMMINILE (4-3-3): Ohrstrom (60' Korpela); Bartoli, Valdezate, Minami, Di Guglielmo; Ciccotti (79' Tomaselli), Troelsgaard, Giugliano (46' Kumagai); Glionna (46' Viens), Giacinti, Haavi (59' Feiersinger)
A disposizione: Sonstevold, Linari, Greggi, Pellegrino Cimo
Allenatore: Alessandro Spugna
FIORENTINA FEMMINILE (4-4-2): Baldi; Faerge, Georgeva (60' Erzen), Agard (82' Spinelli), Toniolo; Janogy (70' Mijatovic), Johannsdottir, Severini (71' Cinotti), Catena; Hammarlund (61' Longo), Boquete
A disposizione: Russo, Tucceri Cimini, Parisi, Lundin
Allenatore: Sebastian De La Fuente
ARBITRO: Valerio Vogliacco
AMMONITE: 21' Bartoli (R); 33' Giugliano (R); 49' Catena (F)
ESPULSE: nessuna

18/05/2024 ore 15:00
SASSUOLO FEMMINILE-JUVENTUS WOMEN 2-3
Marcatori: 30' Echegini (J), 34' Caruso (J), 61' Kullashi (S), 74' Girelli (J), 81' Zamanian Le Loc'h Bakhtiari (Rig.) (S)
SASSUOLO FEMMINILE (4-3-3): Durand; Orsi (72' Zamanian Le Loc'h Bakhtiari), Filangeri, Pleidrup, Philtjens; Mihelic, Pondini, Prugna; Clelland (72' Monterubbiano), Sabatino (59' Kullashi), Beccari
A disposizione: Simon, Santoro, Passeri, Jane, Lonni, Kresche
Allenatore: Gianpiero Piovani
JUVENTUS WOMEN (4-3-3): Peyraud-Magnin; Gama (59' Lenzini), Calligaris (46' Sliskovic), Cascarino, Boattin (46' Cafferata); Echegini, Pelgander, Caruso; Bonansea (73' Garbino), Nystrom, Bragonzi (59' Girelli)
A disposizione: Beerensteyn, Gunnarsdottir, Salvai, Aprile
Allenatore: Paolo Beruatto
ARBITRO: Simone Gavini
AMMONITE: 38' Gama (J); 56' Peyraud-Magnin (J); 71' Bonansea (J); 90+4' Filangeri (S)
ESPULSE: nessuna

Classifica ottenuta dalla somma dei punti della Prima fase più quelli della Poule scudetto.
Prima, seconda e terza classificata vengono ammesse alla Women's Champions League 2024-2025.

VC	NC	PC	GFC	GSC	PtT	GT	VT	NT	PT	GFT	GST	M.I.	
13	0	0	41	8	31	13	10	1	2	33	16	18	
10	1	2	40	12	28	13	9	1	3	25	15	7	
7	2	4	22	17	19	13	5	4	4	20	23	-10	
5	1	7	19	20	20	13	6	2	5	20	21	-16	
4	4	5	19	20	18	13	6	0	7	26	26	-18	

GFC Gol fatti in casa. **GSC** Gol subiti in casa. **STATISTICHE IN TRASFERTA: PtT** Punti in trasferta. **GT** Partite giocate in trasferta. **VT** Partite vinte in trasferta. **NT** Partite pareggiate in trasferta. **PT** Partite perse in trasferta. **GFT** Goal fatti in trasferta. **GST** Goal subiti in trasferta. **M.I.** Media inglese

Giornate e Tabellini

1

GIORNATA

Como Women	1
Napoli Femminile	1
Pomigliano Femminile	0
Sampdoria Femminile	5

Tabellini

17/03/2024 ore 12:30

COMO WOMEN-NAPOLI FEMMINILE 1-1

Reti: 49' Pettenuzzo (Aut.) (N), 69' Del Estal (N)

COMO WOMEN (4-2-3-1): Gilardi; Bergersen Schaathun, Cox (77' Lundorf Skovsen), Lipman, Zanoli; Pastrenge (68' Hilaj), Vaitukaityt?; Picchi (68' Karlernas), Kajan, Monnecchi (60' Skorvankova); Martinovic

A disposizione: Korenciova, Rizzon, Bianchi, Regazzoli, Colombo

Allenatore: Marco Bruzzano

NAPOLI FEMMINILE (4-4-2): Beretta; Pellinghelli, Pettenuzzo, Di Marino (46' Di Bari), Kobayashi; Giacobbo (67' Lazaro Torres Del Molino), Giai (46' Corelli), Gallazzi (87' Kajzba), Chmielinski; Banusic Meredinho (77' Mauri), Del Estal

A disposizione: Fabiano, Veritti, Bertucci, Gianfico

Allenatore: Biagio Seno

ARBITRO: Mattia Nigro

AMMONITE: 35' Giai (N); 45+1' Del Estal (N); 79' Chmielinski (N); 90+1' Hilaj (C)

ESPULSE: nessuno

16/03/2024 ore 12:30

POMIGLIANO FEMMINILE-SAMPDORIA FEMMINILE 0-5

Reti: 24' Rabot (Aut.) (P), 46' Della Peruta V. (S), 67' Della Peruta V. (S), 85' Della Peruta V. (S), 88' Della Peruta V. (S)

POMIGLIANO FEMMINILE (3-5-2): Buhigas; Battistini, Apicella, Caiazzo; Harvey Lynn (84' Novellino), Ferrario, Rabot (70' Szymanowski), Di Giammarino, Fusini (50' Nambi); Ippolito, Arcangeli

A disposizione: Gavillet Vingiani Schettino, Domi Illiano, Manca

Allenatore: Roberto Carannante

SAMPDORIA FEMMINILE (4-3-3): Tampieri; De Rita (79' Heroum), Re, Pisani (82' Marenco), Oliviero; Schatzer, Benoit, Giordano; Baldi (82' Della Peruta T.), Della Peruta V., Cuschieri (89' Nagy)

A disposizione: Tinti, Panzeri, Brustia, Battelani, Fallico

Allenatore: Salvatore Mango

ARBITRO: Felipe Salvatore Viapiana

AMMONITE: 37' Benoit (S); 52' Baldi (S)

ESPULSE: nessuno

2

GIORNATA

Milan Femminile	4
Pomigliano Femminile	0
Sampdoria Femminile	1
Como Women	0

Tabellini

24/03/2024 ore 12:30

MILAN FEMMINILE-POMIGLIANO FEMMINILE 4-0

Reti: 15' Dompig (M), 43' Dompig (M), 47' Ijeh (M), 59' Vigilucci (M)

MILAN FEMMINILE (4-3-3): Giuliani; Piga (58' Vigilucci), Swaby (58' Fusetti), Mesjasz, Bergamaschi; Dubcova, Cernoia, Grimshaw (66' Rubio Avila); Dompig (69' Marinelli), Nadim (65' Asllani), Ijeh

A disposizione: Copetti, Guagni, Mascarello, Donolato

Allenatore: Davide Corti

POMIGLIANO FEMMINILE (3-5-2): Buhigas; Battistini (52' Nambi), Apicella, Caiazzo (78' Domi); Harvey Lynn, Ferrario, Rabot, Di Giammarino (67' Novellino), Fusini; Ippolito (78' Szymanowski), Arcangeli

A disposizione: Gavillet, Vingiani, Schettino

Allenatore: Roberto Carannante

ARBITRO: Jules Roland Andeng

Tona Mbei
AMMONITE: 75' Vigilucci (M)
ESPULSE: nessuno

23/03/2024 ore 12:30
SAMPDORIA FEMMINILE-CO-MO WOMEN 1-0
Reti: 11' Della Peruta V. (S)
SAMPDORIA FEMMINILE (4-3-3): Tampieri; De Rita, Re, Pisani, Oliviero; Schatzer, Benoit, Giordano (75' Heroum); Cuschieri, Della Peruta V., Baldi (70' Della Peruta T.)
A disposizione: Karresmaa, Panzeri, Marenco, Nagy, Brustia, Battelani, Fallico
Allenatore: Salvatore Mango
COMO WOMEN (4-4-2): Korenciova; Lundorf Skovsen (67' Zanoli), Rizzon, Lipman (79' Cox), Bergersen Schaathun; Skorvankova, Picchi, Vaitukaityte (79' Karlernas), Kajan (57' Pastrenge); Sevenius (67' Monnecchi), Martinovic
A disposizione: Gilardi, Bianchi, Regazzoli, Colombo
Allenatore: Marco Bruzzano
ARBITRO: Gabriele Restaldo
AMMONITE: 39' Oliviero (S); 78' Re (S); 80' Bergersen Schaathun (C); 86' Della Peruta V. (S)
ESPULSE: nessuno

3

| Como Women | 1 |
| Milan Femminile | 4 |

| Napoli Femminile | 2 |
| Sampdoria Femminile | 0 |

Tabellini

30/03/2024 ore 18:00
COMO WOMEN - MILAN FEMMINILE 1-4
Reti: 5' Dompig (M), 27' Karlernas (C), 55' Vigilucci (M), 76' Laurent (M), 79' Laurent (M)
COMO WOMEN (4-2-3-1): Korenciova; Bergersen Schaathun, Rizzon, Lipman, Zanoli; Karlernas (83' Hilaj), Pastrenge (70' Vaitukaityt?); Monnecchi (83' Regazzoli), Skorvankova (82' Picchi), Kajan; Martinovic (60' Sevenius)
A disposizione: Gilardi, Liva, Cox, Bianchi
Allenatore: Stefano Maccoppi
MILAN FEMMINILE (4-3-3): Giuliani; Guagni (63' Cernoia), Mesjasz, Piga, Bergamaschi; Vigilucci, Mascarello, Grimshaw (36' Dubcova); Dompig (77' Marinelli), Ijeh (77' Nadim), Asllani (46' Laurent)
A disposizione: Babb, Fusetti, Soffia, Boldrini
Allenatore: Davide Corti
ARBITRO: Lucio Felice Angelillo
AMMONITE: 49' Rizzon (C); 73' Ijeh (M)
ESPULSE: nessuno

30/03/2024 ore 12:30
NAPOLI FEMMINILE-SAMPDORIA FEMMINILE 2-0
Reti: 51' Tampieri (Aut.) (S), 83' Lazaro Torres Del Molino (N)
NAPOLI FEMMINILE (4-3-3): Beretta; Pellinghelli (46' Bertucci,) Pettenuzzo, Di Marino, Kobayashi; Giacobbo (46' Corelli; 90+1' Kajzba), Gallazzi (82' Mauri), Giai; Chmielinski, Del Estal, Banusic Meredinho (82' Lazaro Torres Del Molino)
A disposizione: Fabiano, Di Bari, Veritti, Gianfico
Allenatore: Biagio Seno
SAMPDORIA FEMMINILE (4-1-4-1): Tampieri; De Rita (88' Heroum), Re, Pisani, Oliviero; Benoit (88' Fallico); Cuschieri (72' Lopez Toaquiza), Schatzer, Giordano, Baldi; Battelani (55' Della Peruta T.)
A disposizione: Karresmaa, Panzeri, Marenco, Nagy, Brustia
Allenatore: Salvatore Mango
ARBITRO: Giuseppe Vingo
AMMONITE: 47' Battelani (S); 57' Re (S); 58' Pettenuzzo (N)
ESPULSE: nessuno

4

| Milan Femminile | 3 |
| Napoli Femminile | 2 |

| Pomigliano Femminile | 1 |
| Como Women | 2 |

Tabellini

14/04/2024 ore 15:00
MILAN FEMMINILE-NAPOLI FEMMINILE 3-2
Reti: 45+2' Mascarello (M), 62' Del Estal (N), 64' Bergamaschi (M), 87' Piga (Aut.) (M), 90+2' Dubcova (M)
MILAN FEMMINILE (4-3-3): Babb; Guagni (68' Rubio Avila), Swaby, Piga, Bergamaschi; Cernoia, Mascarello (46' Laurent), Vigilucci; Dompig (90+1' Marinelli), Nadim (46' Dubcova), Ijeh (68' Staskova)
A disposizione: Giuliani, Copetti, Fusetti, Soffia
Allenatore: Davide Corti
NAPOLI FEMMINILE (4-3-3): Beretta; Bertucci (76' Di Bari), Di Marino, Pettenuzzo, Kobayashi; Giacobbo (61' Lazaro Torres Del Molino), Gallazzi, Giai (77' Kajzba); Banusic Meredinho (90+1' Mauri), Del Estal, Chmielinski
A disposizione: Fabiano, Bacic, Veritti, Pellinghelli, Togawa
Allenatore: Biagio Seno
ARBITRO: Gabriele Totaro
AMMONITE: 44' Mascarello (M)
ESPULSE: nessuno

13/04/2024 ore 14:30
POMIGLIANO FEMMINILE-COMO WOMEN 1-2
Reti: 16' Sevenius (C), 18' Arcangeli (P), 68' Sevenius (C)
POMIGLIANO FEMMINILE (4-3-3): Gavillet; Harvey Lynn, Apicella, Caiazzo, Fusini; Rabot (91' Buhigas), Ferrario, Di Giammari-

no (71' Szymanowski); Novellino (77' Manca), Nambi, Arcangeli
A disposizione: Battistini, Vingiani, Corrado, Schettino, Domi, Illiano
Allenatore: Roberto Carannante
COMO WOMEN (4-2-3-1): Gilardi; Bergersen Schaathun, Cox, Rizzon, Zanoli; Hilaj, Pastrenge (58' Karlernas); Lundorf Skovsen (52' Skorvankova), Vaitukaityt?, Monnecchi (75' Picchi); Sevenius (75' Martinovic)
A disposizione: Korenciova, Lipman, Liva, Bianchi, Regazzoli
Allenatore: Stefano Maccoppi
ARBITRO: Gabriele Restaldo
AMMONITE: 64' Hilaj (C); 84' Skorvankova (C); 90+2' Picchi (C)
ESPULSE: nessuno

5

GIORNATA

| Napoli Femminile | 1 |
| Pomigliano Femminile | 1 |

| Sampdoria Femminile | 1 |
| Milan Femminile | 3 |

Tabellini

20/04/2024 ore 15:00
NAPOLI FEMMINILE-POMIGLIANO FEMMINILE 1-1
Reti: 53' Arcangeli (P), 62' Banusic Meredinho (N)
NAPOLI FEMMINILE (4-3-3): Bacic; Bertucci (90+1' Di Bari), Di Marino, Pettenuzzo, Kobayashi; Chmielinski (84' Corelli), Gallazzi, Giai (46' Kajzba); Giacobbo (58' Lazaro Torres Del Molino), Del Estal, Banusic Meredinho
A disposizione: Beretta, Veritti, Pellinghelli, Mauri, Togawa
Allenatore: Biagio Seno
POMIGLIANO FEMMINILE (4-3-3): Gavillet; Harvey Lynn, Apicella, Caiazzo, Fusini; Rabot, Ferrario, Di Giammarino (79' Nambi);

Novellino, Szymanowski, Arcangeli
A disposizione: Buhigas, Battistini, Vingiani, Corrado, Schettino, Domi, Illiano, Manca
Allenatore: Roberto Carannante
ARBITRO: Marco Di Loreto
AMMONITE: 38' Giai (N); 61' Novellino (P); 72' Lazaro Torres Del Molino (N); 87' Ferrario (P); 90+1' Di Bari (N)
ESPULSE: nessuno

21/04/2024 ore 12:30
SAMPDORIA FEMMINILE-MILAN FEMMINILE 1-3
Reti: 45' Dubcova (M), 47' Ijeh (M), 49' Della Peruta T. (S), 80' Ijeh (M)
SAMPDORIA FEMMINILE (4-3-3): Tampieri; De Rita (88' Nagy), Re, Pisani, Oliviero; Schatzer, Benoit (88' Fallico), Giordano (79' Cuschieri); Tatiely, Della Peruta T. (69' Brustia), Baldi (69' Della Peruta V.)
A disposizione: Karresmaa, Panzeri, Heroum, Battelani
Allenatore: Gian Loris Rossi
MILAN FEMMINILE (4-3-3): Giuliani; Guagni (82' Soffia), Dubcova, Piga, Bergamaschi; Cernoia (71' Laurent), Mascarello (81' Rubio Avila), Asllani (60' Vigilucci); Dompig (82' Marinelli), Mesjasz, Ijeh
A disposizione: Babb, Fusetti, Swaby, Arrigoni
Allenatore: Davide Corti
ARBITRO: Edoardo Manedo Mazzoni
AMMONITE: 53' Baldi (S); 54' Bergamaschi (M); 61' De Rita (S); 74' Mascarello (M)
ESPULSE: nessuno

6

GIORNATA

| Napoli Femminile | 1 |
| Como Women | 1 |

| Sampdoria Femminile | 2 |
| Pomigliano Femminile | 2 |

Tabellini

27/04/2024 ore 14:30
NAPOLI FEMMINILE-COMO WOMEN 1-1
Reti: 45' Martinovic (C), 79' Banusic Meredinho (N)
NAPOLI FEMMINILE (4-3-3): Bacic; Pellinghelli, Pettenuzzo, Di Marino, Kobayashi; Giai (50' Chmielinski), Gallazzi, Kajzba (77' Gianfico); Corelli (64' Giacobbo), Del Estal, Banusic Meredinho
A disposizione: Beretta, Di Bari, Veritti, Bertucci, Mauri, Togawa
Allenatore: Biagio Seno
COMO WOMEN (4-2-3-1): Gilardi; Bergersen Schaathun, Rizzon, Cox, Zanoli; Pastrenge (66' Picchi), Hilaj; Monnecchi (44' Martinovic), Skorvankova (90+1' Lundorf Skovsen), Kajan (66' Vaitukaityt?); Sevenius (90' Lipman)
A disposizione: Ruma, Bianchi, Karlernas, Regazzoli
Allenatore: Stefano Maccoppi
ARBITRO: Emanuele Ceriello
AMMONITE: 53' Zanoli (C); 56' Chmielinski (N); 69' Hilaj (C); 81' Martinovic (C); 88' Gianfico (N)
ESPULSE: espulso l'allenatore Biagio Seno (Napoli Femminile)

27/04/2024 ore 12:30
SAMPDORIA FEMMINILE-POMIGLIANO FEMMINILE 2-2
Reti: 6' De Rita (S), 40' Szymanowski (P), 90+1' Baldi (S), 90+4' Novellino (P)
SAMPDORIA FEMMINILE (4-4-1-1): Karresmaa; Brustia (58' Giordano), Pisani, Panzeri, Oliviero; De Rita, Benoit (74' Della Peruta T.), Schatzer (89' Heroum), Cuschieri (74' Baldi); Tatiely (58' Battelani); Della Peruta V.
A disposizione: Tampieri, Nagy, Re, Fallico
Allenatore: Gian Loris Rossi
POMIGLIANO FEMMINILE (4-3-3): Gavillet; Harvey Lynn, Apicella, Caiazzo, Fusini; Rabot, Ferrario, Di Giammarino; Novel-

lino, Szymanowski (89' Nambi), Arcangeli

A disposizione: Caramelli, Battistini, Corrado, Schettino, Domi, Manca
Allenatore: Roberto Carannante
ARBITRO: Giorgio Di Cicco
AMMONITE: 60' Novellino (P); 90+3' Pisani (S)
ESPULSE: nessuno

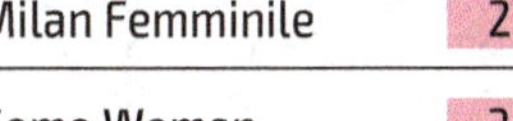

GIORNATA

| Pomigliano Femminile | 2 |
| Milan Femminile | 2 |

| Como Women | 3 |
| Sampdoria Femminile | 1 |

Tabellini

01/05/2024 ore 12:30
POMIGLIANO FEMMINILE-MILAN FEMMINILE 2-2
Marcatori: 5' Mesjasz (M), 52' Mesjasz (M), 73' Szymanowski (P), 88' Rabot (P)
POMIGLIANO FEMMINILE (4-3-3): Gavillet; Novellino, Apicella, Caiazzo, Fusini; Rabot, Ferrario, Di Giammarino (72' Domi); Harvey Lynn (54' Nambi), Szymanowski, Arcangeli
A disposizione: Caramelli, Battistini, Vingiani, Corrado, Schettino, Illiano, Manca
Allenatore: Roberto Carannante
MILAN FEMMINILE (4-3-3): Babb; Guagni (76' Piga), Swaby, Mesjasz, Soffia; Cernoia (70' Arrigoni), Rubio Avila (65' Mascarello), Dubcova; Laurent, Ijeh (65' Staskova), Dompig (70' Marinelli)
A disposizione: Giuliani, Copetti, Fusetti, Cesarini
Allenatore: Davide Corti
ARBITRO: Adolfo Baratta
AMMONITE: 85' Nambi (P)
ESPULSE: nessuna

01/05/2024 ore 15:00
COMO WOMEN-SAMPDORIA FEMMINILE 3-1
Reti: 17' Kajan (Rig.) (C), 46' Karlernas (C), 47' Baldi (S), 69' Karlernas (C)
COMO WOMEN (4-2-3-1): Korenciova; Lundorf Skovsen, Lipman, Cox, Bergersen Schaathun (54' Zanoli); Hilaj (54' Pastrenge), Vaitukaityte; Picchi (84' Bianchi), Karlernas (81' Regazzoli), Kajan (54' Sevenius); Martinovic
A disposizione: Gilardi, Rizzon, Colombo, Monnecchi
Allenatore: Stefano Maccoppi
SAMPDORIA FEMMINILE (4-1-4-1): Karresmaa; Heroum, Pisani, Panzeri, Oliviero; Benoit (76' Cuschieri); Giordano (70' Tatiely), Della Peruta T. (76' Fallico), Schatzer (62' Re), Baldi; Della Peruta V.
A disposizione: Tampieri, Marenco, Nagy, Brustia, Battelani
Allenatore: Gian Loris Rossi
ARBITRO: Alberto Poli
AMMONITE: 16' Karresmaa (S); 37' Lipman (C); 90+2' Zanoli (C)
ESPULSE: nessuno

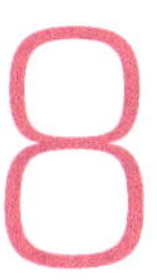

GIORNATA

| Milan Femminile | 1 |
| Como Women | 0 |

| Sampdoria Femminile | 2 |
| Napoli Femminile | 0 |

Tabellini

05/05/2024 ore 15:00
MILAN FEMMINILE-COMO WOMEN 1-0
Marcatori: 27' Soffia (M)
MILAN FEMMINILE (4-3-3): Giuliani; Bergamaschi, Mesjasz, Piga , Soffia (78' Guagni); Cernoia, Mascarello (62' Laurent), Vigilucci; Dompig (78' Nadim), Asllani (62' Rubio Avila), Ijeh (90+4' Swaby)
A disposizione: Copetti, Fusetti, Staskova, Marinelli
Allenatore: Davide Corti
COMO WOMEN (4-2-3-1): Gilardi; Bergersen Schaathun, Rizzon, Cox, Zanoli; Pastrenge (73' Picchi), Hilaj (80' Karlernas); Monnecchi, Skorvankova, Kajan (54' Martinovic); Sevenius
A disposizione: Korenciova, Lipman, Lundorf Skovsen, Bianchi, Regazzoli, Colombo
Allenatore: Stefano Maccoppi
ARBITRO: Francesco Burlando
AMMONITE: 23' Mascarello (M); 35' Zanoli (C); 90+2' Bergamaschi (M)
ESPULSE: nessuna

05/05/2024 ore 12:30
SAMPDORIA FEMMINILE-NAPOLI FEMMINILE 2-0
Reti: 14' Della Peruta V. (S), 25' Della Peruta V. (S)
SAMPDORIA FEMMINILE (4-3-3): Tampieri; Brustia (64' Cuschieri), Pisani, Fallico, Oliviero; De Rita, Re, Giordano; Della Peruta V. (79' Tarenzi), Della Peruta T. (79' Battelani), Baldi (64' Heroum)
A disposizione: Karresmaa, Panzeri, Nagy, Benoit, Tatiely
Allenatore: Gian Loris Rossi
NAPOLI FEMMINILE (4-3-3): Bacic; Di Bari (76' Gianfico), Pettenuzzo, Di Marino, Kobayashi; Chmielinski (76' Bertucci), Gallazzi, Kajzba (46' Lazaro Torres Del Molino); Corelli (59' Giai; 87' Giacobbo), Banusic Meredinho, Del Estal
A disposizione: Beretta, Veritti, Pellinghelli, Mauri
Allenatore: Biagio Seno
ARBITRO: Andrea Zoppi
AMMONITE: 43' Kajzba (N); 52' Brustia (S); 77' Bacic (N); 84' Battelani (S); 90+1' Banusic Meredinho (N); 90+1' Banusic Meredinho (N)
ESPULSE: 90' Banusic Meredinho (N)

| Napoli Femminile | 1 |
| Milan Femminile | 1 |

| Como Women | 2 |
| Pomigliano Femminile | 0 |

Tabellini

12/05/2024 ore 12:30
NAPOLI FEMMINILE-MILAN FEMMINILE 1-1
Marcatori: 11' Gallazzi (Aut.) (N), 84' Chmielinski (N)
NAPOLI FEMMINILE (4-4-2): Bacic; Pellinghelli, Pettenuzzo, Di Marino, Kobayashi; Giacobbo (62' Corelli), Gallazzi, Mauri (63' Giai), Chmielinski; Del Estal, Lazaro Torres Del Molino (72' Gianfico)
A disposizione: Beretta, Di Bari, Veritti, Bertucci, Kajzba, Togawa
Allenatore: Biagio Seno
MILAN FEMMINILE (4-3-3): Giuliani; Bergamaschi (78' Guagni), Piga , Mesjasz, Soffia; Vigilucci, Cernoia, Dubcova (66' Rubio Avila); Asllani (56' Ijeh), Staskova (56' Marinelli), Dom-

pig
A disposizione: Babb, Copetti, Fusetti, Swaby, Arrigoni
Allenatore: Davide Corti
ARBITRO: Giorgio Di Cicco
AMMONITE: 73' Gallazzi (N)
ESPULSE: nessuna

12/05/2024 ore 12:30
COMO WOMEN-POMIGLIANO FEMMINILE 2-0
Marcatori: 53' Martinovic (C), 67' Karlernas (C)
COMO WOMEN (4-2-3-1): Korenciova; Bergersen Schaathun, Rizzon, Lipman, Lundorf Skovsen; Vaitukaityte, Pastrenge (46' Hilaj); Picchi (65' Monnecchi), Karlernas (77' Regazzoli), Skorvankova (72' Bianchi); Martinovic (65' Sevenius)
A disposizione: Gilardi, Zanoli, Liva, Cox
Allenatore: Stefano Maccoppi
POMIGLIANO FEMMINILE (4-3-3): Gavillet; Novellino, Apicella, Caiazzo, Fusini (86' Battistini); Rabot, Ferrario, Di Giammarino (65' Domi); Harvey Lynn (56' Nambi), Szymanowski, Arcangeli
A disposizione: Caramelli, Corrado, Schettino, Manca
Allenatore: Roberto Carannante
ARBITRO: Gioele Iacobellis
AMMONITE: 55' Harvey Lynn (P)
ESPULSE: nessuna

| Pomigliano Femminile | 3 |
| Napoli Femminile | 1 |

| Milan Femminile | 3 |
| Sampdoria Femminile | 1 |

Tabellini

19/05/2024 ore 12:30
POMIGLIANO FEMMINILE-NAPOLI FEMMINILE 3-1
Marcatori: 9' Lazaro Torres Del Molino (N), 43' Ferrario (P), 60' Manca (P), 63' Ferrario (P)
POMIGLIANO FEMMINILE (4-3-3): Gavillet; Battistini (85' Vingiani), Apicella, Caiazzo, Fusini; Rabot, Domi (75' Corrado), Di Giammarino (85' Illiano); Nambi (46' Manca), Ferrario, Arcangeli (49' Schettino)
A disposizione: Caramelli, Harvey Lynn, Novellino
Allenatore: Roberto Carannante
NAPOLI FEMMINILE (4-3-3): Fabiano; Bertucci , Di Bari, Veritti, Pellinghelli (61' Cammarano); Giai (69' D'Angelo), Mauri (46' Langella), Kajzba; Giacobbo (50' Corelli), Lazaro Torres Del Moli-

Classifica

Squadra	Pt	G	V	N	P	GF	GS	PtC	GC
Milan Femminile	41	26	11	8	7	44	30	25	13
Como Women	32	26	9	5	12	30	43	15	13
Sampdoria Femminile	28	26	8	4	14	25	42	14	13
Napoli Femminile	13	26	2	7	17	20	49	10	13
Pomigliano Femminile	12	26	2	6	18	23	65	8	13

LEGENDA STATISTICHE GENERALI: Pt Punti. **G** Partite giocate. **V** Partite vinte. **N** Partite pareggiate. **P** Partite perse. **GF** Gol fatti. **GS** Gol subiti - **STATISTICHE IN CASA: PtC** Punti in casa. **GC** Partite giocate in casa. **VC** Partite vinte in casa. **NC** Partite pareggiate in casa. **PC** Partite perse in casa.

no (46' Gianfico), Togawa
A disposizione: Beretta, Di Marino, Chmielinski
Allenatore: Biagio Seno
ARBITRO: Silvia Gasperotti
AMMONITE: 70' Veritti (N); 81' Corelli (N)
ESPULSE: nessuna

18/05/2024 ore 18:00
MILAN FEMMINILE-SAMPDORIA FEMMINILE 3-1
Reti: 4' Asllani (M), 21' Asllani (M), 74' Re (S), 90+4' Marinelli (M)
MILAN FEMMINILE (4-3-3): Babb (90+1' Copetti); Guagni (69' Soffia), Fusetti (70' Mesjasz), Piga, Bergamaschi; Rubio Avila, Cernoia, Dubcova; Dompig, Asllani (87' Arrigoni), Ijeh (46' Marinelli)
A disposizione: Giuliani, Cesarini, Mikulica, Laurent
Allenatore: Davide Corti
SAMPDORIA FEMMINILE (4-3-3): Tampieri; Brustia (89' Tarenzi), Panzeri, Re, Oliviero; Giordano (57' Nagy), Fallico (57' Benoit), Della Peruta T.; Cuschieri (72' Micheli), Tatiely, Baldi (57' Della Peruta V.)
A disposizione: Karresmaa, Tinti, Marenco, Battelani
Allenatore: Gian Loris Rossi
ARBITRO: Davide Gandino
AMMONITE: 74' Brustia (S); 83' Babb (M)
ESPULSE: nessuno

SPAREGGIO SALVEZZA

Gara di andata

22/05/2024 ore 16:00
TERNANA WOMEN-NAPOLI FEMMINILE 1-2
Reti: 31' Pettenuzzo (N), 72' Labate (T), 90+1' Di Marino (N)
TERNANA WOMEN (3-5-2): Ghioc; Pacioni (81' Lombardo), Quazzico, Di Criscio; Zannini (46' Wagner), Gonzalez Rodriguez, Fusar Poli, Ferrara (46' Tarantino), Vigliucci; Labate, Pirone
A disposizione: Maffei, Santoro, Siejka, Berti, Marenic, Sacco
Allenatore: Fabio Melillo
NAPOLI FEMMINILE (4-4-2): Bacic; Pellinghelli, Pettenuzzo, Di Marino, Kobayashi; Gallazzi (77' Giai), Lazaro Torres Del Molino, Mauri, Chmielinski; Del Estal, Banusic Meredinho (77' Giacobbo)
A disposizione: Veritti, Corelli, Di Bari, Gianfico, Bertucci, Kajzba, Beretta
Allenatore: Biagio Seno
ARBITRO: Samuele Andreano
AMMONITE: 10' Pettenuzzo (N); 57' Quazzico (T)
ESPULSE: nessuna

Gara di ritorno

26/05/2024 ore 16:00
NAPOLI FEMMINILE-TERNANA WOMEN 0-0
NAPOLI FEMMINILE (4-3-3): Bacic; Kobayashi, Di Marino, Veritti, Pellinghelli (90+3' Di Bari); Mauri, Gallazzi (61' Giai), Chmielinski; Del Estal, Banusic Meredinho (61' Giacobbo), Lazaro Torres Del Molino
A disposizione: Bertucci, Kajzba, Gianfico, Corelli, Beretta
Allenatore: Biagio Seno
TERNANA WOMEN (4-2-3-1): Ghioc; Zannini, Pacioni, Di Criscio, Vigliucci; Fusar Poli (90+2' Ferrara), Wagner (90+1' Berti); Labate, Gonzalez Rodriguez, Tarantino (83' Lombardo); Pirone
A disposizione: Maffei, Siejka, Quazzico, Sacco, Santoro, Marenic
Allenatore: Fabio Melillo
ARBITRO: Stefano Milone
AMMONITE: 13' Banusic Meredinho (N); 43' Gonzalez Rodriguez (T); 51' Fusar Poli (T); 53' Pirone (T); 90+4' Giai (N)
ESPULSE: nessuna

Classifica ottenuta dalla somma dei punti della Prima fase più quelli della Poule salvezza.
L'ultima retrocede direttamente in Serie B e la penultima si gioca la permanenza nella massima serie in una gara di playout contro la seconda classificata del campionato cadetto.

VC	NC	PC	GFC	GSC	PtT	GT	VT	NT	PT	GFT	GST	M.I.	
7	4	2	28	17	16	13	4	4	5	16	13	-11	ACM
4	3	6	13	17	17	13	5	2	6	17	26	-20	
4	2	7	10	22	14	13	4	2	7	15	20	-24	
2	4	7	12	18	3	13	0	3	10	8	31	-39	NAPOLI N
2	2	9	16	36	4	13	0	4	9	7	29	-40	POMIGLI

GFC Gol fatti in casa. **GSC** Gol subiti in casa. **STATISTICHE IN TRASFERTA: PtT** Punti in trasferta. **GT** Partite giocate in trasferta. **VT** Partite vinte in trasferta. **NT** Partite pareggiate in trasferta. **PT** Partite perse in trasferta. **GFT** Goal fatti in trasferta. **GST** Goal subiti in trasferta. **M.I.** Media inglese

i 24 record
della Serie A Femminile

Vittorie

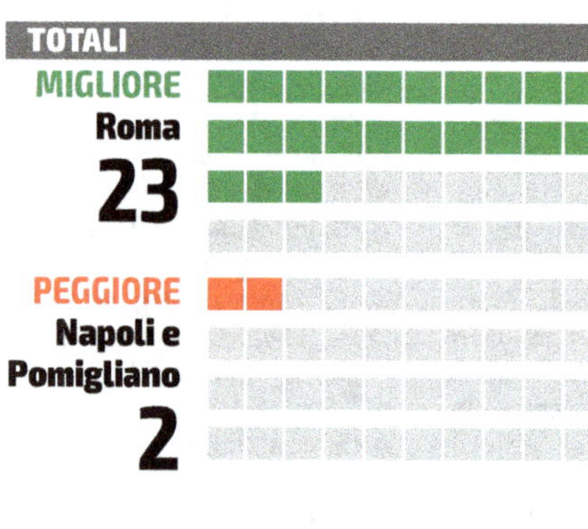

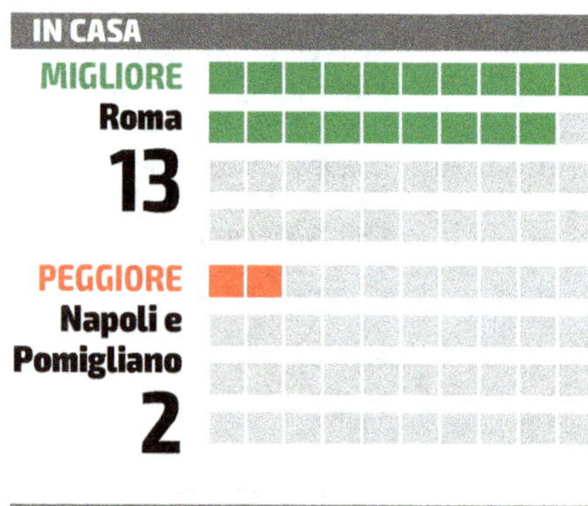

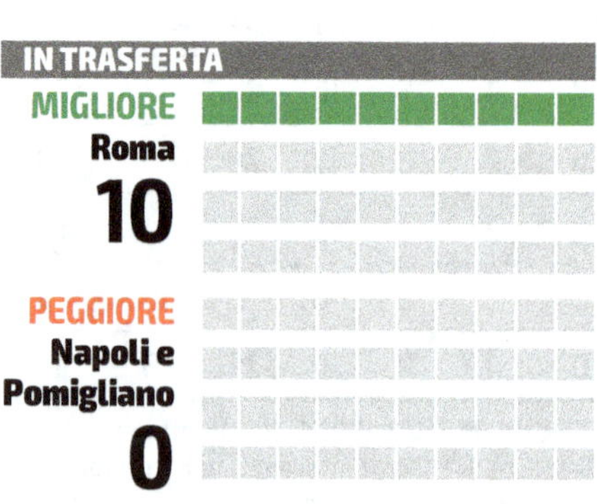

Sconfitte

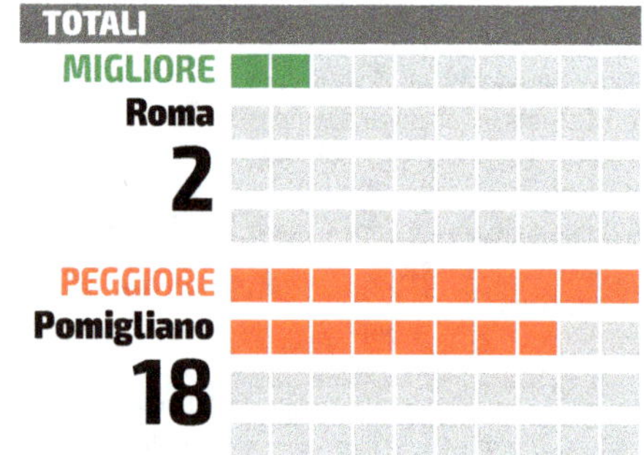

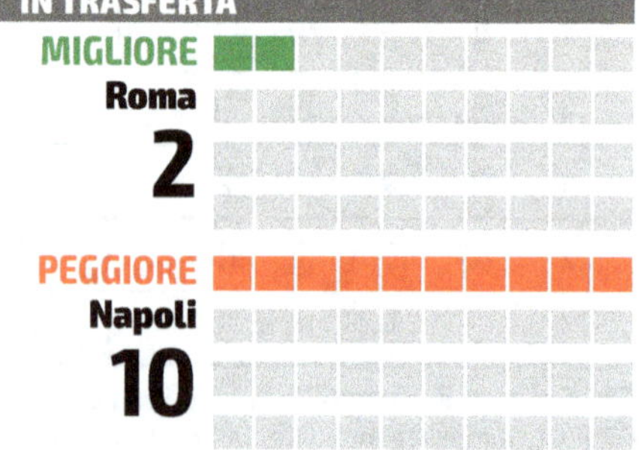

Gol fatti

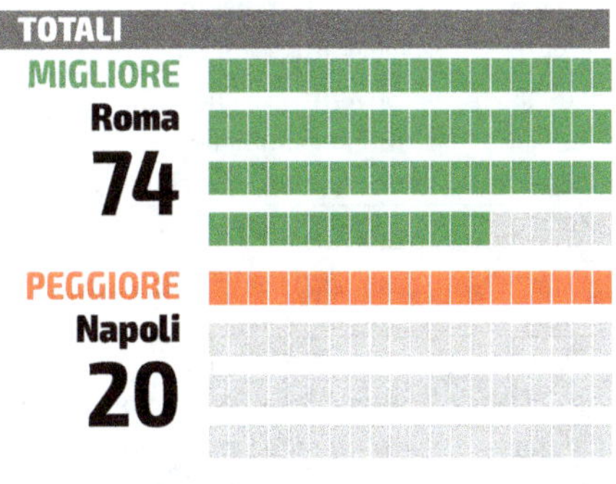

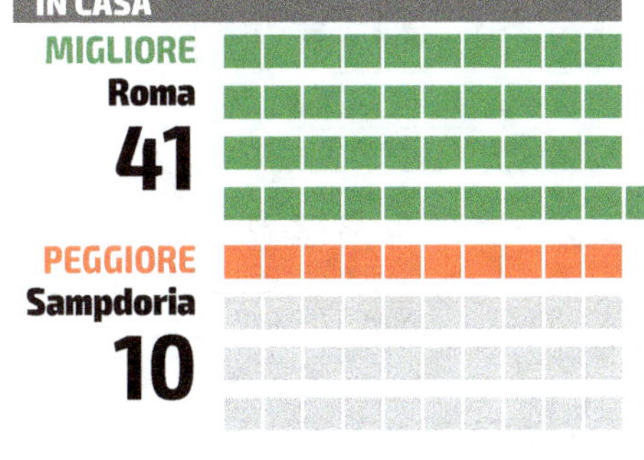

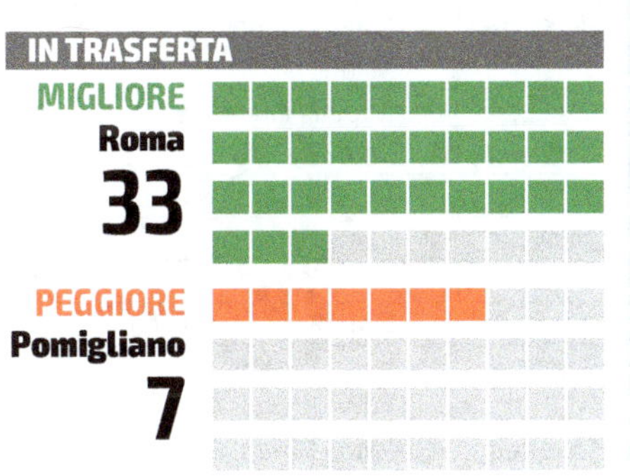

Gol subiti

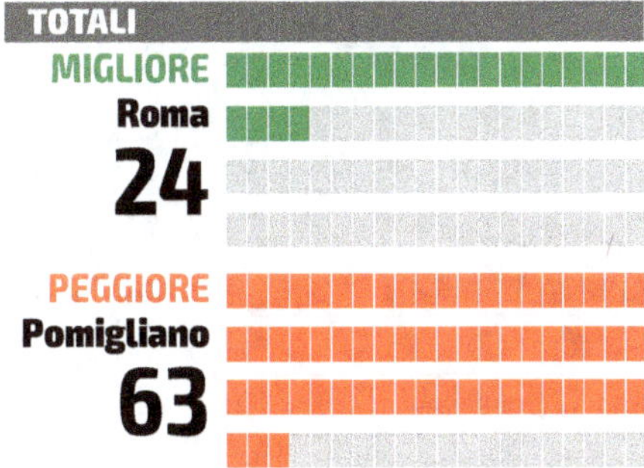

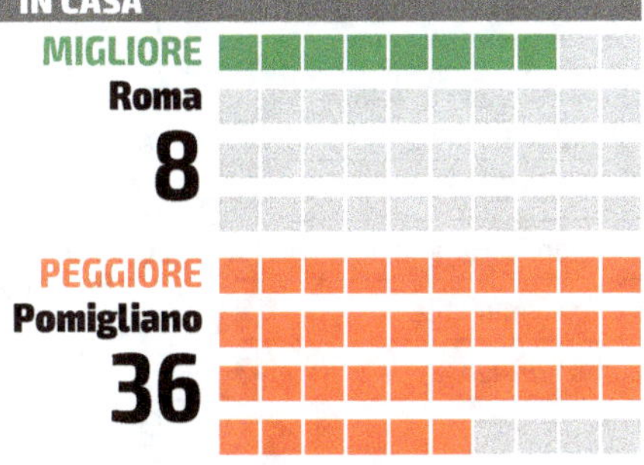

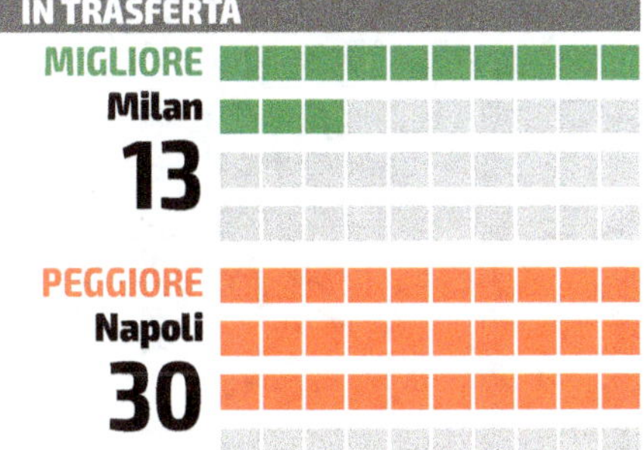

Statistiche
Squadra e Singoli

Goal

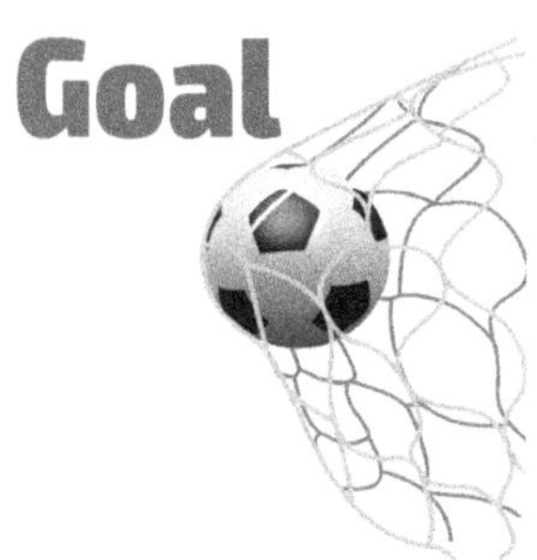

GIOCATORI IN RETE

Squadra

Roma Femminile	**16**
Juventus Women	**14**
Milan Femminile	**14**
Inter Women	**12**
Fiorentina Femminile	**11**
Pomigliano Femminile	**11**
Sassuolo Femminile	**11**
Sampdoria Femminile	**10**
Napoli Femminile	**9**
Como Women	**8**

CLASSIFICA CANNONIERI

	Nome	Cognome	Squadra	Goal
1	Evelyne	Viens	Roma Femminile	13
2	Valentina	Giacinti	Roma Femminile	12
3	Cristiana	Girelli	Juventus Women	11
4	Jennifer	Echegini	Juventus Women	10
5	Manuela	Giugliano	Roma Femminile	10
6	Veronica	Boquete	Fiorentina Femminile	9
7	Lina	Magull	Inter Women	9
8	Lana	Clelland	Sassuolo Femminile	9
9	Agnese	Bonfantini	Inter Women	8
10	Lindsey K.	Thomas	Juventus Women	8
11	Victoria M.	Della Peruta V.	Sampdoria Femminile	8
12	Michela	Catena	Fiorentina Femminile	7
13	Madelena	Janogy	Fiorentina Femminile	7
14	Michela	Cambiaghi	Inter Women	7
15	Lineth	Beerensteyn	Juventus Women	7
16	Arianna	Caruso	Juventus Women	7
17	Elena	Linari	Roma Femminile	7
18	Loreta	Kullashi	Sassuolo Femminile	7
19	Daniela	Sabatino	Sassuolo Femminile	7
20	Zsanett Bernadet	Kajan	Fiorentina Femminile/ Como Women	6
21	Julia	Karlernas	Como Women	6
22	Melania	Martinovic	Como Women	6
23	Julia A.	Grosso	Juventus Women	6
24	Kosovare	Asllani	Milan Femminile	6
25	Chante M.	Dompig	Milan Femminile	6
26	Andrea	Staskova	Milan Femminile	6
27	Elisa M.	Del Estal	Napoli Femminile	6
28	Saki	Kumagai	Roma Femminile	5
29	Chiara	Beccari	Sassuolo Femminile	5
30	Oona	Sevenius	Como Women	4
31	Dominika	Skorvankova	Como Women	4
32	Miriam	Longo	Fiorentina Femminile	4
33	Haley	Bugeja	Inter Women	4
34	Elisa	Polli	Inter Women	4
35	Annamaria	Serturini	Roma Femminile/ Inter Women	4

	Nome	Cognome	Squadra	Minuti Giocati	Goal	Minuti/ Goal
1	Victoria Marie	Della Peruta V.	Sampdoria Femminile	558	8	70
2	Jennifer	Echegini	Juventus Women	738	10	74
3	Cristiana	Girelli	Juventus Women	1339	11	122
4	Lindsey Kimberly	Thomas	Juventus Women	1017	8	127
5	Evelyne	Viens	Roma Femminile	1660	13	128
6	Lina	Magull	Inter Women	1158	9	129
7	Madelena	Janogy	Fiorentina Femminile	916	7	131
8	Valentina	Giacinti	Roma Femminile	1665	12	139
9	Lana	Clelland	Sassuolo Femminile	1347	9	150
10	Melania	Martinovic	Como Women	976	6	163
11	Annamaria	Serturini	Roma Femminile/ Inter Women	654	4	164
12	Kosovare	Asllani	Milan Femminile	1061	6	177
13	Zsanett Bernadet	Kajan	Fiorentina Femminile/ Como Women	1095	6	183
14	Manuela	Giugliano	Roma Femminile	1947	10	195
15	Loreta	Kullashi	Sassuolo Femminile	1385	7	198
16	Laura	Feiersinger	Roma Femminile	803	4	201
17	Agnese	Bonfantini	Inter Women	1690	8	211
18	Daniela	Sabatino	Sassuolo Femminile	1543	7	220
19	Veronica	Boquete	Fiorentina Femminile	2022	9	225
20	Andrea	Staskova	Milan Femminile	1388	6	231
21	Michela	Cambiaghi	Inter Women	1678	7	240
22	Elisa	Polli	Inter Women	967	4	242
23	Lineth	Beerensteyn	Juventus Women	1709	7	244
24	Haley	Bugeja	Inter Women	1026	4	257
25	Chiara	Beccari	Sassuolo Femminile	1290	5	258
26	Julia	Karlernas	Como Women	1633	6	272
27	Elisa Mateu	Del Estal	Napoli Femminile	1645	6	274
28	Julia Angela	Grosso	Juventus Women	1648	6	275
29	Elena	Linari	Roma Femminile	1948	7	278
30	Michela	Catena	Fiorentina Femminile	1977	7	282
31	Arianna	Caruso	Juventus Women	1987	7	284
32	Miriam	Longo	Fiorentina Femminile	1161	4	290
33	Chante Mary D.	Dompig	Milan Femminile	1758	6	293
34	Sofia	Cantore	Juventus Women	1250	4	313
35	Emelyne Ann-E.	Laurent	Milan Femminile	1251	4	313
36	Lucia	Di Guglielmo	Roma Femminile	1371	4	343
37	Oona	Sevenius	Como Women	1465	4	366
38	Saki	Kumagai	Roma Femminile	2019	5	404
39	Dominika	Skorvankova	Como Women	1632	4	408
40	Giada	Greggi	Roma Femminile	1658	4	415
41	Cristina S. N.	Tatiely	Sampdoria Femminile	1788	4	447

Gialli

SQUADRE CON PIÙ AMMONITI

Napoli Femminile	49
Como Women	42
Sampdoria Femminile	41
Fiorentina Femminile	37
Pomigliano Femminile	34
Milan Femminile	33
Juventus Women	29
Inter Women	28
Sassuolo Femminile	28
Roma Femminile	25

I GIOCATORI PIÙ AMMONITI

	Nome	Cognome	Ruolo	Squadra
8	Cecilia	Re	CEN	Sampdoria Femminile
7	Alma	Hilaj	CEN	Como Women
6	Emma	Severini	CEN	Fiorentina Femminile
6	Valentina	Bergamaschi	DIF	Milan Femminile
6	Martina	Di Bari	DIF	Napoli Femminile
5	Kaja	Erzen	DIF	Fiorentina Femminile
5	Martina	Toniolo	DIF	Fiorentina Femminile
5	Pauline	Peyraud-Magnin	POR	Juventus Women
5	Marta	Mascarello	CEN	Milan Femminile
5	Paloma	Lazaro Torres	ATT	Napoli Femminile
5	Cristina S.	Tatiely	ATT	Sampdoria Femminile
5	M. Luisa	Filangeri	DIF	Sassuolo Femminile
4	Julia	Karlernas	CEN	Como Women
4	Dominika	Skorvankova	CEN	Como Women
4	Liucija	Vaitukaityte	CEN	Como Women
4	Martina	Zanoli	DIF	Fiorentina F./Como W.
4	Henrietta	Csiszar	CEN	Inter Women
4	Ghoutia	Karchouni	CEN	Inter Women
4	Flaminia	Simonetti	CEN	Inter Women
4	Arianna	Caruso	CEN	Juventus Women
4	Julie	Piga	DIF	Milan Femminile
4	Alice	Corelli	ATT	Napoli Femminile
4	Valentina	Gallazzi	CEN	Napoli Femminile
4	Tecla	Pettenuzzo	DIF	Napoli Femminile
4	Virginia	Di Giammarino	CEN	Pomigliano Femminile
4	Debora	Novellino	DIF	Pomigliano Femminile
4	Alice	Benoit	CEN	Sampdoria Femminile
4	Aurora	De Rita	DIF	Sampdoria Femminile

Rossi

SQUADRE CON PIÙ ESPULSI

Juventus Women	2
Fiorentina Femminile	1
Milan Femminile	1
Napoli Femminile	1
Pomigliano Femminile	1
Roma Femminile	1
Sassuolo Femminile	1
Como Women	0
Inter Women	0
Sampdoria Femminile	0

I GIOCATORI PIÙ ESPULSI

	Nome	Cognome	Ruolo	Squadra
1	Marina	Georgeva	DIF	Fiorentina Femminile
1	Barbara	Bonansea	ATT	Juventus Women
1	Sara Bjork	Gunnarsdottir	CEN	Juventus Women
1	Emelyne Ann-E.	Laurent	ATT	Milan Femminile
1	Marija	Banusic Meredinho	ATT	Napoli Femminile
1	Gaia	Apicella	DIF	Pomigliano Femminile
1	Elisa	Bartoli	DIF	Roma Femminile
1	Erika	Santoro	DIF	Sassuolo Femminile

Serie A Femminile

L'Organigramma

Federica Cappelletti Presidente
Elena Turra Vicepresidente
Stefano Braghin, Alessandro Terzi Consiglieri

Il formato

Il formato della Serie A femminile 2023-2024 prevede due fasi.

Nella prima fase le dieci squadre partecipanti si affronteranno in un girone all'italiana con partite di andata e ritorno per un totale di diciotto giornate.

Nella seconda fase le prime cinque compagini in graduatoria accederanno a una poule scudetto con in palio il titolo di Campione d'Italia (prima classificata) e l'ammissione alla Women's Champions League 2024-2025 (prima, seconda e terza classificata), mentre le altre cinque prenderanno parte a una poule salvezza al termine della quale l'ultima retrocederà direttamente in Serie B e la penultima si giocherà la permanenza nella massima serie in una gara di playout contro la seconda classificata del campionato cadetto.

In entrambe le poule, le squadre, portando in dote i punti ottenuti nella prima fase, si incontreranno in un girone all'italiana con partite di andata e ritorno per ulteriori dieci giornate complessive (due turni di riposo a testa).

Il regolamento

Il regolamento prevede tre punti per la vittoria, uno per il pareggio e nessuno per la sconfitta. In caso di arrivo di due o più squadre a pari punti per stilare la graduatoria si terrà conto nell'ordine dei seguenti criteri: punti negli scontri diretti, differenza reti negli scontri diretti, differenza reti generale e reti realizzate in generale. In caso di parità anche nel numero totale dei gol segnati si procederà al sorteggio.

L'albo d'oro

Edizione	Federazione organizzatrice	Campione d'Italia
1968	FICF	Genova
	UISP	Bologna CF
1969	FICF	ACF Roma
	UISP	Bologna CF
1970	FFIGC	Gommagomma Meda
	FICF	Real Torino
1971	FFIGC	Brevetti Gabbiano Piacenza
	FICF	ACF Real Juventus
1972	FFIUAGC	Gamma 3 Padova
1973	FFIGC	Gamma 3 Padova
	FICF	ACF Milano
1974	FFIUGC	Falchi Astro Montecatini
1975	FIGCF	USF Milan
1976	FIGCF	Valdobbiadene
1977	FIGCF	Diadora Valdobbiadene
1978	FIGCF	Jolly Catania

Edizione	Federazione organizzatrice	Campione d'Italia
1979	FIGCF	Lazio CF 1975 Lubiam
1980	FIGCF	Lazio CF 1975 Lubiam
1981	FIGCF	Alaska Gelati Lecce
1982	FIGCF	Alaska Gelati Lecce
1983	FIGCF	Alaska Gelati Lecce
1984	FIGCF	Alaska Trani 80
1985	FIGCF	Sanitas Trani 80
1985-86	FIGCF	Despar Trani 80
1986-87	FIGC-LND	Lazio CF
1987-88	FIGC-LND	Lazio CF
1988-89	FIGC-LND	Campania G.B. Giugliano
1989-90	FIGC-LND	Reggiana Refrattari Zambelli
1990-91	FIGC-LND	Reggiana Refrattari Zambelli

Edizione	Federazione organizzatrice	Campione d'Italia
1991-92	FIGC-LND	Milan 82 Salvarani
1992-93	FIGC-LND	Reggiana Refrattari Zambelli
1993-94	FIGC-LND	Torres Fo. S
1994-95	FIGC-LND	Agliana
1995-96	FIGC-LND	Verona Gunther
1996-97	FIGC-LND	Modena
1997-98	FIGC-LND	Modena
1998-99	FIGC-LND	ACF Milan
99-2000	FIGC-LND	Torres Fo. S
2000-01	FIGC-LND	Torres Fo. S
2001-02	FIGC-LND	Ruco Line Lazio
2002-03	FIGC-LND	Foroni Verona
2003-04	FIGC-LND	Foroni Verona
2004-05	FIGC-LND	Poliplast Bardolino Verona
2005-06	FIGC-LND	Fiamma Monza
2006-07	FIGC-LND	Bardolino Verona

Edizione	Federazione organizzatrice	Campione d'Italia
2007-08	FIGC-LND	Centropose Bardolino Verona
2008-09	FIGC-LND	Bardolino Verona
2009-10	FIGC-LND	Torres
2010-11	FIGC-LND	Torres
2011-12	FIGC-LND	Torres
2012-13	FIGC-LND	Torres
2013-14	FIGC-LND	Brescia
2014-15	FIGC-LND	AGSM Verona
2015-16	FIGC-LND	Brescia
2016-17	FIGC-LND	Fiorentina
2017-18	FIGC-LND	Juventus
2018-19	FIGC	Juventus
2019-20	FIGC	Juventus
2020-21	FIGC	Juventus
2021-22	FIGC	Juventus
2022-23	FIGC	AS Roma
2023-24	FIGC	AS Roma

Gli arbitri

I numeri   94 Arbitri   173 Assistenti arbitrali

nome	cognome	distretto
Commissione Arbitri Nazionale Serie C		
Responsabile		
Maurizio	**Ciampi**	Roma 1
Componenti		
Nicola G.	**Ayroldi**	Molfetta
Luca	**Banti**	Livorno
Gianluca	**Cariolato**	Legnago
Fabio	**Comito**	Torino
Pasquale	**Rodomonti**	Teramo
Arbitri		
Claudio G.	**Allegretta**	Molfetta
Andrea	**Ancora**	Roma 1
Jules Roland	**Andeng Tona Mbei**	Cuneo
Samuele	**Andreano**	Prato
Lucio Felice	**Angelillo**	Nola
Albert Ruben	**Arena**	Torre del Greco
Adolfo	**Baratta**	Rossano
Andrea	**Bordin***	Bassano del Grappa
Giorgio	**Bozzetto**	Bergamo
Francesco	**Burlando**	Genova
Mattia	**Caldera**	Como
Andrea	**Calzavara**	Varese
Matteo	**Canci***	Carrara
Enrico	**Cappai**	Cagliari
Domenico	**Castellone**	Napoli
Luigi	**Catanoso**	R. Calabria

nome	cognome	distretto
Gianluca	**Catanzaro**	Catanzaro
Ermes F.	**Cavaliere**	Paola
Matteo	**Centi**	Terni
Erminio	**Cerbasi**	Arezzo
Emanuele	**Ceriello**	Chiari
Luca	**Cherchi**	Carbonia
Filippo	**Colaninno**	Nola
Antonino	**Costanza**	Agrigento
Valerio	**Crezzini**	Siena
Luca	**De Angeli**	Milano
Michele	**Delrio**	Reggio Emilia
Francesco	**D'Eusanio**	Faenza
Giorgio	**Di Cicco**	Lanciano
Dario	**Di Francesco**	Ostia Lido
Marco	**Di Loreto**	Terni
Antonio	**Di Reda**	Molfetta
Abdoulaye	**Diop**	Treviglio
Aleksandar	**Djurdjevic**	Trieste
Mattia	**Drigo**	Portogruaro
Marco	**Emmanuele**	Pisa
Emanuele	**Frascaro***	Firenze
Simone	**Galipò**	Firenze
Davide	**Gandino**	Alessandria
Mauro	**Gangi**	Enna
Silvia	**Gasperotti**	Rovereto
Simone	**Gauzolino**	Torino
Simone	**Gavini**	Aprilia
Enrico	**Gemelli***	Messina

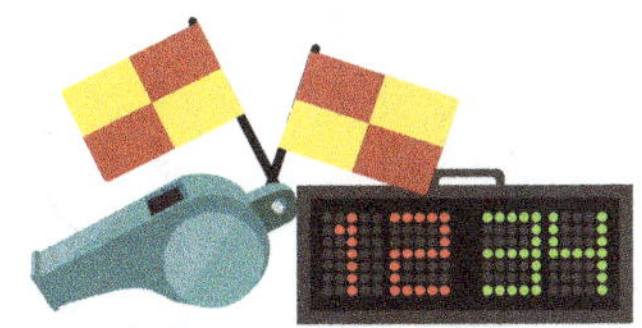

nome	cognome	distretto
Filippo	**Giaccaglia**	Jesi
Edoardo	**Gianquinto**	Parma
Enrico	**Gigliotti**	Cosenza
Gianluca	**Grasso***	Ariano Irpino
Gioele	**Iacobellis**	Pisa
Alfredo	**Iannello**	Messina
Domenico	**Leone**	Barletta
Ettore	**Longo***	Cuneo
Roberto	**Lovison***	Padova
Fabio Rosario	**Luongo**	Napoli
Lorenzo	**Maccarini**	Arezzo
Dario	**Madonia***	Palermo
Giuseppe Maria	**Manzo**	Torre Annunziata
Maria	**Marotta**	Sapri
Leonardo	**Mastro-domenico**	Matera
Edoardo M.	**Mazzoni**	Prato
Stefano	**Milone**	Taurianova
Domenico	**Mirabella**	Napoli
Katerina	**Monzul'**	Torino
Giuseppe	**Mucera**	Palermo
Stefano	**Nicolini**	Brescia
Mattia	**Nigro**	Prato
Fabrizio	**Pacella**	Roma 2
Marco	**Peletti**	Crema
Mario	**Perri**	Roma 1

nome	cognome	distretto
Valerio	**Pezzopane**	L'Aquila
Alberto	**Poli**	Verona
Fabrizio	**Ramondino**	Palermo
Gianluca	**Renzi**	Pesaro
Gabriele	**Restaldo**	Ivrea
Carlo	**Rinaldi**	Bassano del Grappa
Giuseppe	**Rispoli***	Locri
Gabriele	**Sacchi**	Macerata
Eugenio	**Scarpa**	Collegno
Gabriele	**Scatena**	Avezzano
Bogdan N.	**Sfira***	Pordenone
Alessandro	**Silvestri**	Roma 1
Simone	**Taricone***	Perugia
Gabriele	**Totaro**	Lecce
Niccolò	**Turrini***	Firenze
Mattia	**Ubaldi**	Roma 1
Cristiano	**Ursini**	Pescara
Giorgio	**Vergaro**	Bari
Felipe S.	**Viapiana**	Catanzaro
Giuseppe	**Vingo**	Pisa
Daniele	**Virgilio**	Trapani
Valerio	**Vogliacco**	Bari
Francesco	**Zago**	Conegliano
Andrea	**Zanotti**	Rimini
Andrea	**Zoppi**	Firenze

* Nessuna designazione per gare del Campionato di Serie A Femminile 2023-2024

Datasport
a tappe

La Storia di un miglioramento costante nella gestione della comunicazione sportiva

2023/2024 Si esplorano nuovi media, nuove organizzazioni, nuovi prodotti sempre più periferici e locali partendo da una base dati globale sempre più grande.
Obiettivo di periodo: l'adozione del Tempo Effettivo nel Calcio nei pro e negli amatori.

2022 novembre Inizia l'era della Intelligenza Artificiale. Le competenze si amplificano e coinvolgono grandi gruppi di persone ognuno competente nel suo ruolo e diventa difficile competere con il video sempre più dedicato e frammentato.

2021/2023 Ricerca di nuovi approcci di un settore editoriale allo sbando.

2019/2020 Introduzione di un nuovo concetto di comunicazione del calcio in modo trasversale nei mezzi, nel tempo e nei media. Soddisfazione di tutti i bisogni informativi per tutte le classi di età, per tutti i diversi interessi, per qualunque mezzo utilizzato per la consultazione.

2018/2019 Datasport nuova versione e progetto "Una persona in ogni Stadio".

2017 Parte su www.datasport.it la pubblicazione, modello YearBook americano, dei dati di tutte le partite dalla Serie A ai Dilettanti e alle Giovanili, Live con i dati statistici, progetto che vanta numerosi tentativi di imitazione.

2016/2024 Pubblicazione di 20 almanacchi Yearbook con i dati di tutta la stagione, dalla Serie A maschile e femminile alla Primavera passando Serie C e Serie D, sia in carta sia in ebook. Importante la dedizione al Progetto di Matteo Pifferi, di Alberto Rossi e delle competenze grafiche di Antonella Colucci.

2016 Partecipazione alle Olimpiadi di Rio de Janeiro con innovazioni e approfondimenti tecnici non presenti sino ad allora con uso di computer di ultima generazione che hanno piantato in asso tutti e tre gli inviati.

2012 Partecipazione alle Olimpiadi di Londra con innovazioni e approfondimenti tecnici, video ed internet, non presenti sino ad allora. Storie umane e di colore dalle Olimpiadi. Storie degli atleti italiani raccontate dal campo di gara a cura di Guido Di Santo.

2006 Campionato Mondiale di Calcio di Germania: interviste audio in diretta sul sito internet con uso di un telefonino per la connessione e di un apparato tecnico appositamente predisposto per la registrazione. Prime parole di Andrea Pirlo, capitano della squadra italiana campione del Mondo, in diretta in italiano su un sito internet.

2004 Partecipazione alle Olimpiadi di Atene con innovazioni e approfondimenti tecnici non presenti sino ad allora.

2000 Presa in carico come 1°Editore del

manuale di Fantacalcio di Riccardo Albini, Alberto Rossetti e Benedetta. Prima uscita assoluta del concetto Fantasy Football già presente negli Stati Uniti.

2000 RAI Televideo, introduzione del concetto notiziario aggiornato sulle attività delle squadre con il resoconto dalle sedi di allenamento.
Partecipazione alle Olimpiadi di Sydney con innovazioni e approfondimenti tecnici. Intervista a Mohamed Ali.

1996 Analisi tecnica per la modifica del regolamento del calcio FIFA (passaggio al portiere, 10 raccattapalle, recupero, barella in campo, Tabellone per comunicare il tempo da recuperare, ecc.). Presentatore del Progetto: Paolo Casarin.

1995 1° luglio Pubblicazione del primo numero di Datasport.it, sito e notiziario internet su tutto lo sport italiano Sei mesi prima del leader della comunicazione sportiva italiana.

1994 Primo sito di notizie di calcio Datasport.it - Internet World Wide Web con server a Rende (CS) collegato con il mondo attraverso una T-Bone Motorola. Promotore attività informatiche Francesco Marrara. Primo esempio di clouds collegati con il mondo senza rendercene conto.

1992/1998 Collaborazione con AIA e FIGC con l'analisi tecnica delle partite e delle prestazioni degli arbitri. Presidente Gianni Petrucci e designatore degli arbitri Paolo Casarin.

1990 Rilevazione Statistica in diretta di tutte le partite del Campionato Mondiale di Calcio Italia '90 - Prima assoluta mondiale. Abbiamo insegnato al mondo che anche il gioco del calcio poteva essere registrato, analizzato e valutato.

1990 Banca Dati FIFA di tutti i giocatori, squadre e partite giocate nei gironi eliminatori e nei gironi finali durante i campionati Mondiali di Calcio dal 1930 al 1986.

1988 Coppa dei Sogni Gazzetta dello Sport a cura di Alessandro De Calò, Paolo Condò, Stefano Bizzotto e Fabio Bianchi, Da un'idea di Enrico Maida e la realizzazione tecnica di Luciano Menghi Responsabile del primo database di dati e notizie (Tesaurus) della RCS e Giacomo Zordan, prezioso e antesignano informatico di Datasport.

1988 Inizio della trasmissione 'Tutto Basket' condotta da Giorgio Micheletti - gestione in tempo reale di tutti i dati del campionato italiano di Serie A.

1987/1989 Redattore insieme a Bruno Talamonti di 'Tutto il Calcio Minuto per Minuto' con conduttori Roberto Bortoluzzi e Massimo De Luca. Incremento delle informazioni sulle partite di Serie C e valorizzazione dei campionati non di Serie A sulla schedina del Totocalcio, detta la Sisal ideata da Massimo Della Pergola successivamente collaboratore di Datasport per i Sistemi da giocare dai tabaccai.

1987 Inizio della trasmissione 'Qui Studio a Voi Stadio' ideata da Ruggero Muttarini e Paolo Romani - gestione informatica e editoriale dei dati sportivi con incremento esponenziale del ricavo pubblicitario televisivo per una trasmissione della domenica pomeriggio.

1986 Raccolta delle statistiche sulla Serie B, ndividuali e di squadra.

1986/2008 Gestione domenicale della pagina 201 di RaiTelevideo con l'introduzione del concetto di risultato in tempo reale dalla Serie A alla D, gestione di 14 campionati in contemporanea. Direttore Giorgio Cingoli, redattori Donatella Scarnati, Paolo Petruccioli, Mauro Mosconi, Guido Fumarola.

1985 1° settembre. Raccolta delle Statistiche individuali e di squadra della Serie A. Gestione del paginone centrale della Gazzetta dello Sport con tutti i dati del Campionato Riferimento preziosissimo per tutti gli appassionati.

Yearbook dei Campionati di Calcio 2023/24

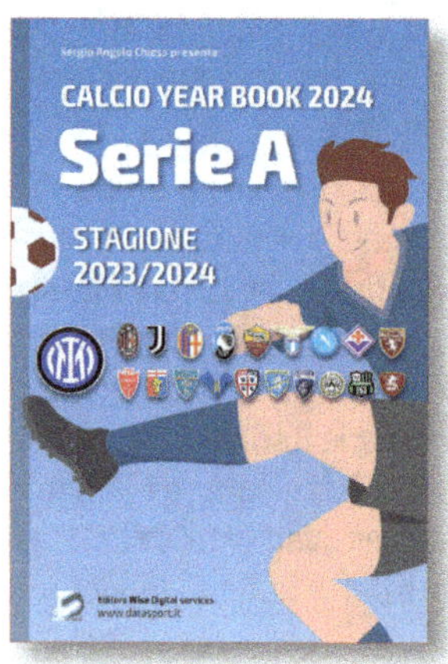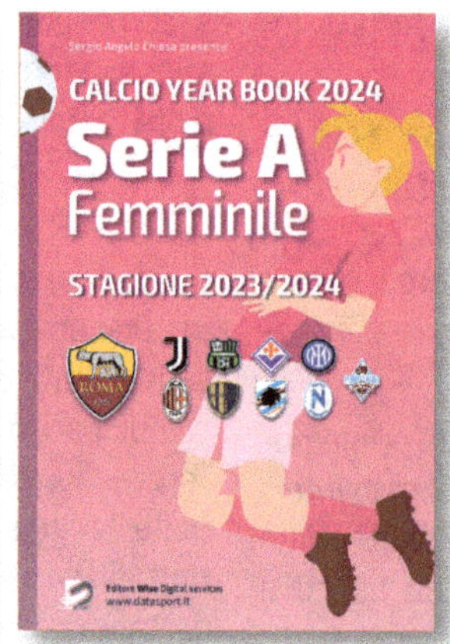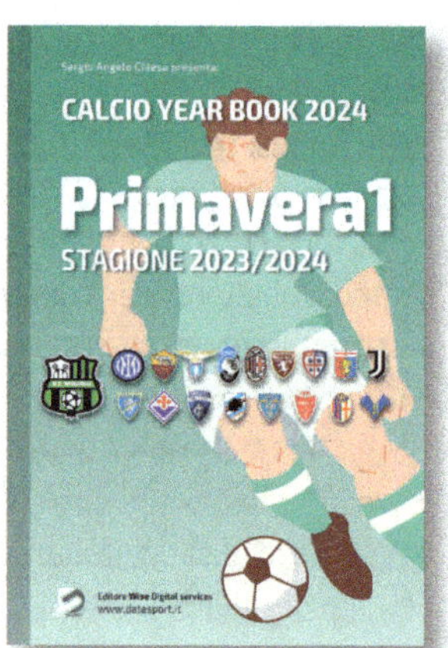

Disponibili su Amazon.it